PRAISE FOR PREVIOUS BOOKS
BY NORTIN M. HADLER

Worried Sick

"*Worried Sick* is for anyone who wants to make wise decisions about how to care for themselves and their loved ones. Dr. Hadler lucidly reveals the expensive tests that determine little and the quick fixes that boost nothing but cost to point the way toward a health system that we can't afford not to have."
—Scott Simon, National Public Radio, author of
Pretty Birds and *Windy City*

"Case by case, drug by drug, test by test, and procedure by procedure, Hadler exposes the excesses, the unjustified costliness, and the ineffectiveness of the present medical scene. He presents a proposal for a health-care insurance system that will increase the health of the nation, provide only effective care, and reduce costs. All self-funded employers must read, absorb, and install Hadler's well-founded ideas."
—Clifton K. Meador, M.D., author of *A Little Book of Doctors'*
Rules, *Med School*, and *Symptoms of Unknown Origin*

"Dr. Hadler . . . is a longtime debunker of much that the establishment holds dear. . . . Reviewing the data behind many of the widely endorsed medical truths of our day, he concludes that most come up too short on benefit and too high on risk to justify widespread credence. . . . Raise[s] serious questions."
—*New York Times*

"Challenging conventional medical wisdom, [Hadler] advises a healthy skepticism about the benefits of drugs, routine tests, and many common medical procedures. . . . Educate[s] [readers] on being far better health-care consumers. . . . [A] provocative look at the U.S. medical system."
—*Library Journal*

"To change unrealistic expectations about longevity or lives without pain or illness bucks vested interests, but that is what Hadler does. . . . He knows that the changes he proposes are a long shot, but when people demand that medicine stop doing unnecessary things well, reform becomes possible. Recommended."
—*Choice*

Rethinking
AGING

Nortin M. Hadler, M.D.

Rethinking
AGING

Growing Old and Living Well in
an Overtreated Society

The University of North Carolina Press   Chapel Hill

Library of Congress Cataloging-in-Publication Data
Hadler, Nortin M.
Rethinking aging : growing old and living well
in an overtreated society / Nortin M. Hadler.
p. ; cm.
Includes bibliographical references and index.
ISBN 978-0-8078-3506-7 (cloth : alk. paper)
1. Older people — Medical care — United States. 2. Older people —
United States — Psychology. 3. Health behavior — United States. I. Title.
[DNLM: 1. Health Services for the Aged — United States. 2. Aged —
psychology — United States. 3. Health Behavior — United States. 4. Health
Promotion — methods — United States. 5. Inappropriate Prescribing —
United States. 6. Social Conditions — United States. WT 31]
RA564.8.H335 2011   362.1084'6 — dc22   2011006663
15 14 13 12 11   5 4 3 2 1

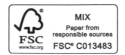

MIX
Paper from
responsible sources
FSC® C013483

Rethinking Aging is published as Carol S. Hadler and I mark the forty-sixth anniversary of our wedding. We have altered the complexion of our careers but not their focus; Carol is a brilliant practicing psychotherapist. We have not altered our commitment to living our lives together as fully as possible for as long as is fated. She is my mentor and soul mate. This book is a statement of my dedication to her.

It is also a statement of our dedication to our children, Jeffrey and Elana; their spouses; and our grandchildren, Eli, Maia, Lucy, Noe, Theo, and Oliver. It is our fervent hope that they will find many pathways open to them in life, that they will have the fortune and fortitude to travel more than one with a degree of fulfillment, that they will never travel without loving and being loved, that they will know the comfort of community, and that they will arrive at age eighty-five able to look back and smile.

CONTENTS

FIGURES AND TABLES

FIGURES

TABLES

PREFACE
ROUNDING WITH MURRAY

Childhood instills notions of aging. There are always the "old" in the room, nearby or on the periphery. Sometimes they're the loving old, the beloved old, the crotchety old, even the wise old. Always the old are different through the eyes of the child—people other than just adults, such as parents. Old to the child is an abstraction.

Not for me. I learned gerontology at my father's knee.

My father was the baby in a family that emigrated from Shepatovka, Ukraine, fin de siècle and settled in Mattapan, a neighborhood of Boston. I know little of the next forty years, mainly a few big-date facts. He was the valedictorian of Boston Latin, which brought an automatic admission to Harvard or MIT; he chose the former. As an undergraduate, he supported himself digging Boston's transit system and working in his father's tailor shop. Against all odds, he was admitted to Harvard Medical School and graduated in 1929. This is not an abridged history; it's nearly all we were to know. It fell on him to support his parents in the deepening Depression. One of his brothers argued that New York City offered more opportunities than Boston. My father did a year of internship at King's County Hospital in Brooklyn and opened his general practice in the Bronx in 1930, catering to a working-class population. He married my mother a decade later with the expressed intention of having a son to send back to Harvard Medical School with the advantages he never enjoyed. I am that son.

I grew up very close to my father. I made house calls with him starting in grade school. He arranged for my first job in a hospital before I was a teenager. I worked in medical facilities nearly every weekend and every summer until college. All the time, I learned about my father's perceptions and projections regarding medicine in the 1950s and about his dreams. Realize that this long predates Medicare. He was called to many a house to attend to a frail older patient who was often part of an extended family. The "fee" for his service was paid more often in gratitude than in cash. My father was a light in the haze of these patients' frailty. Included in these peregrinations were frequent visits to Sanger's Nursing Home, a proprietary facility with many hundreds of beds in a dingy multistory building in midtown Manhattan, where he served as the physician of record. I watched my father's eyes and posture as he ministered to the illnesses that plagued his decrepit and frail patients. I carry his gaze to the bedside to this day.

Decades later found me strutting down the hallowed halls of the University of North Carolina, living the future my father had wished on me. He remained in New York, unwilling to retire. For a decade, he owned and operated a thirty-bed nursing home in a small city up the Hudson River from New York City. He loved the details of its management and the interactions with the local physicians concerning the care of their patients. He went out of his way to know every patient, both medically and personally. And he loved to relate all of this to me.

Regulatory change put an end to such small institutions, but not to my father's calling to work in that milieu. As I intimated, we never knew his age. He was an octogenarian when he assumed a post as a house physician in a large nursing home in the Bronx, where he rotated night call. That means that at least one night a week, he slept in the institution at the beck and call of the nursing staff. I was at *his* beck and call about the clinical challenges he recognized those nights. One 3:00 A.M. call was about a very old patient with low blood sodium, which provoked a lengthy discussion of the implications and its treatment—causing him to return to medical textbooks with the determination of a driven medical student.

Another late-night call led my father to query why his patients were all on a two-gram sodium diet. He appreciated well-prepared food and was disturbed that his patients were forced to eat a diet that seemed unnecessarily unpalatable. It was not clear to me whether any of his patients did or could voice their displeasure. I pointed out that most of them were on fluid pills for their fluid retention or hypertension, so that restricting salt intake to this degree was probably unnecessary and a throwback to a time when medicine had little in the way of appealing pharmaceutical alternatives. My father was troubled by this explanation — not its validity, but its implications. I asked if he wanted to prove me wrong, a challenge that set him back on his heels. This was twenty-five years ago, when there were no Institutional Review Boards to pass on the ethics of clinical investigation; clinicians were held responsible to their conscience and to review by peers. So I designed a randomized trial of prescribing a "no added salt" regular diet (about a four-gram sodium diet) to half his patients and continuing the far-more-restricted two-gram sodium diet for the other half. I instructed my father as to the data he was to collect (weight, blood chemistries, clinical outcomes such as death, etc.) and then forgot about this entire enterprise.

A year later, he called and asked me what he should do with the data. Helping him with the analysis, the preparation of the scientific paper, and its submission for publication is a wonderful and colorful memory that I won't belabor. He knew it was accepted for publication and that the paper would be accompanied by a laudatory editorial by one of the pioneers in gerontology, Eugene Stead. My father died before the actual publication.

Hadler, Morris H. The lack of benefit of modest sodium restriction in the institutionalized elderly. *Journal of the American Geriatrics Society* 1984; 32 (3): 235–36.

With one paper, his only paper, he changed the dietary prescription for the institutionalized elderly and taught his son the last of his invaluable lessons. It colors my practice, my life, and this book. This is not simply a dietary prescription; it is a value-laden proclamation. Not only is the last breath to be valued, but the last smile is to be equally valued, even if it is only assumed and not observable.

I do not know if my father had read William Shakespeare's Sonnet 73. I suspect he had.

That time of year thou mayst in me behold
When yellow leaves, or none, or few, do hang
Upon those boughs which shake against the cold,
Bare ruin'd choirs, where late the sweet birds sang.
In me thou seest the twilight of such day
As after sunset fadeth in the west,
Which by and by black night doth take away,

Death's second self, that seals up all in rest.
In me thou see'st the glowing of such fire
That on the ashes of his youth doth lie,
As the death-bed whereon it must expire
Consumed with that which it was nourish'd by.
  This thou perceivest, which makes thy love more strong,
  To love that well which thou must leave ere long.

ACKNOWLEDGMENTS

In parlance, doctor and physician are synonyms for individuals licensed to practice medicine. I am very proud to bear these titles, but I impute far more to them than their connotations of credentialing and licensure. Doctor is a Latin noun derived from *doceō*, to teach. Physician is from the French *physicien*, a natural philosopher. There is more to being a physican than teaching natural philosophy. These are titles that promise trustworthiness and demand professionalism. The titles demand the exercise of moral philosophy. No one has captured this better than the Persian physician Avicenna, who wrote the following near the turn of the eleventh century.

THE MORNING PRAYER OF THE PHYSICIAN

O God, let my mind be ever clear and enlightened. By the bedside of the patient let no alien thought deflect it. Let everything that experience and scholarship have taught it be present in it and hinder it not in its tranquil work. For great and noble are those scientific judgments that serve the purpose of preserving the health and lives of Thy creatures.

Keep far from me the delusion that I can accomplish all things. Give me the strength, the will, and the opportunity to amplify my knowledge more and more. Today I can disclose things in my knowledge which yesterday I would not yet have dreamt of, for the Art is great, but the human mind presses on untiringly.

In the patient let me ever see only the man. Thou, All-Bountiful One, hast chosen me to watch over the life and death of Thy creatures. I prepare myself now for my calling. Stand Thou by me in this great task, so that it may prosper. For without Thine aid man prospers not even in the smallest things.

Rethinking Aging is my fifteenth book, my fourth for a general audience. I am ever so grateful for a life and a career that allow me to be part of this tradition, and for an editor, David Perry, and his colleagues at UNC Press that help me serve this ethic.

Rethinking
AGING

1

ENLIGHTENED AGING

We all grapple with the greater meaning of death. Philosophers, theologians, and poets have been recruited to the task for eons. I have no special insights as to why we must die or what might follow, nor is my personal philosophy causing me to write this book. But we must die.

Aging, dying, and death are no longer solely the purview of philosophers and clerics. Many biological and epidemiological theories of aging have been articulated. Some are even testable theories, and many have been tested. The result is an informative science. We still have much to learn and many a theory that eludes testing, but the product of all this science is a body of information that has much to say to anyone today who wants to reflect on aging, dying, and death. This book is anchored on this body of information. Beyond reflection, aging, dying, and death have arrived at center stage in realpolitik at the urging of economists and for public-policy considerations given the needs of the burgeoning population of elderly.

Aging, dying, and death are not diseases. Yet they are targets for the most egregious marketing, disease mongering, medicalization, and overtreatment. This book is written to forewarn and arm the reader with evidence-based insights that promote informed medical and social decision making. All who have the good fortune to be healthy enough to confront the challenges of aging need such insights. Otherwise they are no match for the cacophony of broadcast media pronouncing the scare of the week or miracle of the month; pandering magazine articles; best-selling books pushing "angles" of self-interest; and the ubiquitous marketing of pharmaceuticals and alternative potions, poultices, and chants. All are hawking "successful aging" and "long life" as if both were commodities. We awaken every day to advice as to better ways to eat, think, move, and feel as we strive to live longer and better. We are bombarded with the notion of risks lurking in our bodies and in the environment that need to be reduced at all cost. Life, we are told, is a field that is ever more heavily mined with each passing year.

There are places on the globe where life is a literal minefield. There are others where it is a figurative minefield. The latter are places where a ripe old age is the fate of a lucky few, unconscionably only a few. Those places usually have as common denominators inadequate water and sewer facilities, unstable political structures, and dire poverty. They are a reproach to the collective conscience. However, I am writing this book for those of us fortunate enough to reside in the resource-advantaged world, countries that have crossed the epidemiological watershed so that it's safe to drink the water. For us, death before our time is not a fact of life; it's a tragedy. For us, a ripe old age is not a will-o'-the-wisp; it's likely. And this happy and fortunate circumstance has almost nothing to do with what we eat, with our potions and pills, or with our metaphysical beliefs, and it has very little to do with the ministrations of the vaunted "health-care" systems that we underwrite. This will become disconcertingly, even painfully, clear in the chapters that follow.

For now, we need to understand how fortunate we really are. Figure 1 displays U.S. longevity curves. The most recent curve that is available is based on census data that is a decade old. That bears witness to the challenges of finding out who is still alive and when, and at what age, the decedent died. Furthermore, the mathematical equations involved are very sensitive to small changes in age-specific death rates, particularly at the older age groups, when relatively few survive. The curves become more accurate in retrospect. Nonetheless, the message is obvious. Through the twentieth century, the likelihood of becoming an octogenarian increased greatly; the likelihood of becoming a nonagenarian barely budged, if at all. The idealized curve for our species is rectilinear; it is nearly flat because all would survive until their eighty-fifth birthday, more or less, when the curve dives as all die suddenly.

Figure 1 is more than the foundation for this book. It is a celebration of our time in the resource-advantaged world. Ours is not our grandparents' longevity, not even our parents' longevity. A "ripe old age" is no longer a literary device. We know how old one is when one is "ripe": one is an octogenarian. To anchor our notions of aging and our notions of dying in

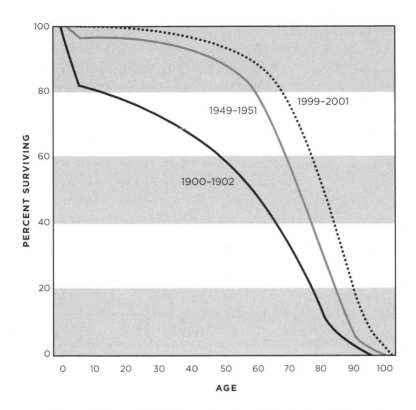

Figure 1. Changes in U.S. longevity rates during the twentieth century. The survival curves over the twentieth century have become increasingly rectangular. This trend is obvious and dramatic prior to 1950. More and more, we are likely to become octogenarians, at which point the curves are increasingly vertical. (U.S. Public Health Service, *National Vital Statistic Reports*, vol. 57, no. 1, August 5, 2008)

any other timetable is irrational. Once I am an octogenarian, the issue is no longer longevity but the quality of the life of the aged. I don't care how many diseases I have once I'm an octogenarian, or which of the many proves my reaper; I want to rejoice in the arriving at a ripe old age and know pleasure in the life of the aged.

Hence, "saving" or prolonging the life of an octogenarian is not a very useful goal. Those who live beyond their eighties can count themselves lucky, though seldom fortunate. Nonagenarians and centenarians, the "old-old," are few and often forlorn. We know something of the biology of dying, enough to encourage venture capitalists to fund biotechnology enterprises seeking a molecular solution. Maybe, someday, there will be a molecular solution to the timing of a ripe old age. Don't hold your breath. This book discounts that possibility.

In my most recent books, I addressed the health concerns of the working-age population. *The Last Well Person: How to Stay Well Despite the Health-Care System* (2004) focuses on medicalization and on Type II Medical Malpractice. Medicalization is reframing ordinary predicaments of life so that they are viewed as diseases. Type II Medical Malpractice is the doing of the unnecessary, even if it is done well. There are myriad examples of the untoward consequences of medicalization. As for Type II Medical Malpractice, it's a scourge. My next book, *Worried Sick: A Prescription for Health in an Overtreated America* (2008), picks up both themes where the first book left off and points to the formulation of rational health-care reform. It was followed by *Stabbed in the Back: Confronting Back Pain in an Overtreated Society* (2009). In that work, I use the experience of low back pain to explore how the context in which backache is suffered, rather than the intensity of pain or its biology, determines the illness experience. Low back pain has spawned flawed health, disability, and compensation-indemnity schemes that are object lessons for health-care reform.

Rethinking Aging: Growing Old and Living Well in an Overtreated Society will take these ideas further, but my target here is not informing the general public about medicalization and Type II Medical Malpractice in order to influence the direction of health-care reform. Neither am I focusing on the population that is traditionally considered "working age." Rather, I am addressing those who are approaching their later decades or have already entered them in order to arm them with the wisdom to question the advice they are receiving from all quarters and to help them conceptualize graceful and successful aging. Seldom will tradition, common sense, religious counsel, and personal fortitude prove a match for the medicalizing of everyday ailments. "Risk factors" abound, and we are told that every risk factor must be addressed—regardless of the benefit of treatment or lack thereof. We are told that every untoward personal challenge needs a biomedical explanation and a biomedical solution, or perhaps an alternative therapy. This book will arm you with the need and the ability to ask, "Does any of this really matter to me?" I want you to be able to make informed medical decisions. I want you to live out the last decades of your allotted fourscore and five as successfully, satisfyingly, and comfortably as possible, unfettered by worrisome notions of health promotion and unnecessary or harmful forms of disease management.

These last decades encompass the last years of gainful employment, the challenge of fulfillment in retirement, and the challenge of dying. It is apparent from Figure 1 that for prior generations of Americans, the interval between the end of gainful employment and the grave was brief. Today, it is not. In designing this book, I was tempted to divide it into three sections: the decade as an aged worker (fifty-five to sixty five), the decade of unfettered active life (sixty-six to seventy-five), and the last decade. However, the sequence is far from inviolate and the timing highly variable. So the chapter that addresses the challenges of being an aged worker pertains whether you're sixty or eighty, and so on. Furthermore, the chapters are not meant to represent passages, a procession from stage to stage. It is possible to be frail but not decrepit or frail and yet an aged worker. The chapters do not denote stations in life. They are important aspects of life that need to be understood, even savored.

Reading with a Prepared Mind

Rethinking Aging is neither a textbook of geriatric medicine nor yet another screed of the "Secrets to Good Health" genre. It is an exercise in logical positivism. In many of the chapters that follow, I employ object lessons to teach how one might make informed medical decisions in the various contexts that are relevant as one negotiates the challenges to health after sixty. Many of these object lessons are powerful because they illustrate errors in reasoning, mistaken beliefs, or misinformation. In some, the errors in reasoning are promulgated by purveyors who serve agendas other than the welfare of the patient. As a result, there is a sheen to *Rethinking Aging* that might be misinterpreted as "doctor bashing." That is neither my intent nor my proclivity. We are all advantaged by the fact that the vast majority of physicians are bright, well trained, and well intended. I know this to be so because I have been privileged for nearly half a century to work among these physicians as colleague, mentor, and consultant. However, the American physician in particular is faced with enormous constraints that compromise ethical behavior—perverse constraints on their time wielded by reimbursement schemes. We can hope that a new institution of medicine will soon supersede one that is ethically bankrupt. Until then, it is crucial that all people who need to be or become patients have a prepared mind. Patients must maintain control of the diagnostic and therapeutic processes. In order to do so, they must be capable of asking about the potential benefits and risks, be willing to demand a detailed answer, and be prepared to actively listen to the answer. It is to this end that I've written *Rethinking Aging*, and it is to this end that I offer these object lessons.

Even Methuselah Died

Many may want to dismiss my discussion above. After all, Aunt Fannie or Uncle Bill lived to ninety-six, and Uncle Bill smoked and loved his doughnuts. Some want to argue that it's all a matter of genes. This book will disabuse you of any such notion. Many genetic traits can conspire to cut short our lives: familial breast or colon cancers, exceptionally high cholesterol, and others. But longevity is not heritable. The reason Aunt Fannie and Uncle Bill made it beyond a ripe old age is stochastic; that is, they are lucky statistical outliers. You have no better chance of being a nonagenarian than if Aunt Fannie or Uncle Bill were not in your family.

Many will regard this as counterintuitive. After all, so many of the patriarchs of the Old Testament were really old. The Judeo-Christian-Islamic tradition holds these old men up as tantamount to gold standards. Longevity is treated as a sign of purposefulness, if not holiness. The Old Testament offers up Abraham, Moses, and that statistical outlier for the ages, Methuselah, the grandfather of Noah, whose age at death is usually translated as 969 years. Some scholars choose a different Sumerian dialect for translation or convert to lunar years and come up with an age closer to eighty-five — exceptional, not too shabby for the time of the Great Flood, and not fatuous, as is 969. We, the residents of the modern resource-advantaged world, are likely to live as long as Methuselah really did. The question I think we need to ask, however, is not simply how can we gain assurance that we will live eighty-five years but can we aspire to be purposeful and self-assured for eighty-five years?

Foreknowledge of the time of one's death would be a heavy burden, not a blessing. Furthermore, if a world without death becomes a world without birth, the specter is bleak and joyless. Rather, for the Judeo-Christian-Islamic tradition and many polytheistic traditions, death is inevitable, and the imponderability of its imperative is assuaged with notions of an afterlife.

The idealized human survival curve has no infant mortality: we all live to eighty-five only to die on our eighty-fifth birthday. Figure 1 is impressive for the fact that survival curves in the United States in the twentieth century are trending toward this ideal. But the curve has a ways to go, and

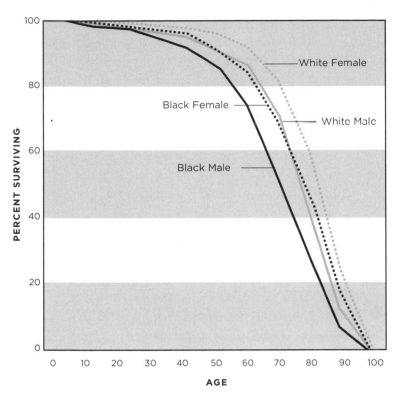

Figure 2. Gender and racial disparities in U.S. longevity rates.
The analysis of the 1999–2001 data illustrated in Figure 1 discerns impressive
gender and racial disparities, illustrated here. (U.S. Public Health Service,
National Vital Statistic Reports, vol. 57, no. 1, August 5, 2008)

the curve for the United States has further to go toward the rectilinear
ideal than that for nearly every other of our peers in the developed world.
True, in America obesity, tobacco, high cholesterol, a health-adverse diet,
inactivity, and so forth are contributing factors. And there is the suggestion that the particular makeup of our society is to blame. Figure 2 shows
the racial and gender discrepancies in the most recent American survival
curves. It's easy to jump to the conclusion that being a black man in America automatically subtracts five years from one's life expectancy. We have
been pummeled with these inferences for so long and so intensively that
they are part of the accepted wisdom. They are not entirely wrong, but
nearly so.

In fact, the list of health-adverse behaviors and cardiovascular risk factors accounts for about 20 to 25 percent of one's mortal hazard — that is,
the years one falls short of a ripe old age. Furthermore, the mortal hazard

inherent in these risk factors is not linear; you have to push the limits to pay this price. Just a little above whatever the "expert" consensus is for normal health behavior du jour imparts little if any hazard.

The remainder of a person's mortal hazard, the bulk of it, relates to the circumstance of community. Beware if you are uncomfortable in your socioeconomic status; faced with a job you hate and have no options; poor; stigmatized in the pecking order; faced with uncertainties as to your future; or ostracized, alone, or lonely. These are some of the attributes of one's ecosystem that chip away at longevity. With the exception of infant mortality, it makes no difference what continent one's ancestors hail from.

All of this is in place before sixty-five, and after sixty-five it all plays out. Much of this was known to the sages of old, even to the authors of the Old Testament:

> The days of our years among them are seventy years
> and if, with special attributes of strength and power,
> eighty years. (Psalm 90, usually attributed to Moses)

2

THE GOLDEN YEARS

This chapter and several that follow have an existential gloss: love, life, and death. But it is only a gloss. Generations of authors have offered up their philosophies, observations, preconceptions, prejudices, and metaphysical beliefs under a rubric such as successful aging, aging well, and the like. Some of this literature is sophomoric, some is quackery, much is self-serving, and much is simply fatuous. I have no inclination to review or even highlight that which I place in these categories. However, some is elegant, eloquently broadening the reader's own personal philosophy. And some is scientific, applying the results of systematic studies to cause one to rethink preconceived notions. I am sorely tempted to try my hand at the eloquently broadening genre; hopefully, a little of such will insinuate into these chapters. But my strength as an author and educator is in this last category.

Our concern in this chapter is the health of those over sixty who are well. We know they are well because they tell us they are well. We know they are well because they tell us they are well despite, or regardless of, or even because of, the biologic imperatives of being over sixty.

All have a burden of disease. "Disease" is a term I use to designate anatomical and biochemical alterations from what would be considered "normal" in midlife. In my terminology, the symptoms that can be ascribed to "disease" by a physician are the "illness." Some diseases are unusual at any age, like leukemia. But there are some that would be abnormal in youth but are so common after sixty that to be spared them is abnormal. Hence, there is a burden of disease that we all earn with each passing year. This is one of the messages of the next chapter, where we will discuss the nonspecificity of so many findings on screening tests. By sixty, some "diseases" are so normal that we dare not call them diseases, like graying or thinning hair—or do we? Illnesses are never normal, even if they are common. The ability to ascribe a particular illness to a definable disease is imperfect at all ages; this inability is commonplace in the elderly.

All have to cope with personal predicaments. We experience many unpleasant symptoms intermittently throughout life. No one escapes heartburn or heartache, headache or eye strain, back pain or knee pain, diarrhea or constipation, or more—at least no one escapes for long. Usually, we cope with such symptoms on our own. These I term predicaments. For some predicaments, we decide to turn to doctors, in which case the symptoms are our illness. The degree to which we can cope on our own is dependent on the context in which we experience the predicament. Aging is its own context.

All are learning to cope with the notion of their own mortality.

All are bombarded, day in and day out, by warnings and forewarnings related to their health. All listen to the scare of the week with one ear and the miracle of the month with the other. We learn that life is a minefield and that so many vendors are willing to purvey their special way through to the other side. Day in and day out, we encounter pills licensed by the Food and Drug Administration (FDA) for prescription or for over-the-counter purveyance. Potions and salves, dietary constraints and dietary supplements, surgical remedies, pillows and mattresses, and more are on the modern therapeutic menu. This can't be avoided or ignored thanks to concerted efforts to whet our appetites by the media, by marketers, by disease mongers, by the purveyors of beliefs, and by sectarian practitioners of every ilk. After all, there is no greater market for all of this than the population currently over sixty. This is the population that controls the greatest personal wealth the industrialized world has ever seen. There is a gold mine under all that gray hair.

Nearly all have health insurance; for all over sixty-five, it is federally underwritten. Coverage is legislated; what is covered is the result of pressures brought to bear on the Medicare administration. Pressures from lobbyists are powerful enough, but it is the pressure brought by common sense that can most easily overwhelm any scientifically based push-back. We will discuss in the next chapter how common sense has forced Congress to mandate that Medicare underwrite mammography despite the contravening science. Common sense is not temporally or geographically common and is seldom sense, but it is always highly susceptible to marketing influences.

All know people who are patients, and some know people their age who suffered terminal illnesses.

Despite this litany, most people over sixty tell us they are well. None are oblivious to all the background health noise in their bodies or in their lives more generally. Some manage to blithely ignore it all; for others, ignoring takes a concerted effort. If you ask people over age fifty to define successful aging, the majority consider good health an essential component. This is followed by psychological factors, social roles and activities, finances, social relationships, and neighborhood.[1] None of these components is readily defined by those of us who are the observers and commentators, nor should we assume that our presuppositions pertain to any group of aging adults, let alone any individual in that group.[2] This chapter is designed to arm all with the epistemology to carry on as well persons for as long as that is reasonable — just as the next chapter is designed to arm all with the epistemology to confront the demands of screening to save their lives.

Carrying Baggage

Social inequalities burden people who are in their older decades at least as much as they did earlier in life. This burden goes well beyond purchasing power. This is dramatic even in Norway, despite its egalitarian ideology and a national health service. People with a higher education live substantially longer than those with a basic education.[3] The effect of social inequalities on health and longevity is magnified the greater the disparity across the population. In the Whitehall II Study, over 10,000 men and women employed in the British civil service were enrolled at age thirty-five to fifty-five and followed for nearly twenty years. People who had worked in lower civil-service grades aged more quickly in terms of their sense of well-being, physical capacity, and disease measures.[4]

One's position on the socioeconomic gradient prior to retirement is the major determinant of one's health in later life and one's longevity. This relationship holds across twenty-two European countries.[5] It also pertains to the gradient of disability across the socioeconomic spectrum in the United States.[6] True, some of the malevolence of social inequalities results from health-adverse behaviors such as smoking or morbid obesity.

But health-adverse behaviors explain only a fraction of the effect.[7] More malevolent are the mortal hazards that lurk in our neighborhood, in our self-actualization, in our wealth or lack thereof, in the stability of our income stream, in our family structure, and in our intimate relationships.[8] There is no reason to assume that any particular influence or combination of influences pertains to a given individual.[9] The secrets to longevity are in the fine structure of human ecology. There is every reason to argue that these are the secrets to the health of the public, to population health going forward.[10]

But are these also the secrets to improving the outcome and outlook for those who have already survived sixty years in their microecological niche? Or are all the cows out of the barn?

Resilience

In the mid-twentieth century, the temporal gap between "retirement" and death was narrow; all the cows were undoubtedly out of the barn. It was so narrow that it drove the construction of facilities dedicated to the compassionate shepherding of elderly persons through the final transitions of life soon after the completion of productive, interactive living.

In the twenty-first century, the cows are munching cud in their stalls. The definition of "retirement" has blurred and the interval between retirement and death has widened—both dramatically. Today, people spend more time in retirement than in childhood and adolescence. Resources and recourses for retirees that seemed appropriate in the middle of the twentieth century hardly pertain to the longevity of today. This has fostered a research agenda that lives under such rubrics as "positive aging," "active aging," "body/retirement satisfaction," or even "mental health in later life." It is an exercise in teasing elements appropriate to the older-age population out of the "socioeconomic status" construct. Community-dwelling people over age sixty-five value having/maintaining physical health and functioning, leisure and social activities, mental functioning and mental activity, and social relationships and contacts.[11] For a younger person, having/maintaining physical health and functioning along with mental functioning and activity are more likely to be taken for granted and supplanted by aspects of employment. The value of leisure and social activities coupled with social relationships and contacts is less age dependent. Social cohesiveness is essential for the years after sixty to be "golden." A growing and compelling scientific literature bears witness to the importance of community and interpersonal networks. We will return to this prerequisite for successful aging at the end of this chapter because it is far more amenable to intervention and control than the other components.

Promoting and Maintaining Physical Health

The last assertion—that one is more likely to promote physical health by attention to social cohesiveness than by attention to human biology—is counterintuitive. We awaken daily to alarms about the epidemics of obesity and type 2 diabetes and all the other drums beating impending doom. For elderly people, the din is even greater: osteopenia, flu, dementia, strokes, heart failure, and so much more are breathing down their backs. And for every darkening shadow there are diagnostic tests, screenings for risk, and treatments galore. The doctor is the gatekeeper who keeps these gates open, and monies flow from Medicare to keep the paths greased. America's elderly know the numbers associated with each of the acronyms that foretell their fate: BMI, HbA1c, BP, LDL, HDL, and BMD, to list the commonplace. And America's elderly swallow the prescribed remedies, often many simultaneously, to bring their laboratory numbers to heel. America's elderly are hell bent to be normal. They assume the swallowing of pills and their attendant adverse effects are either a price well paid or, more likely, a component of the new definition of "normal." America's elderly lead the world in this exercise and are the envy of their peers elsewhere for their tenacity and wherewithal.

It's all so sad. They are on a fool's errand.

It's OK to Be Overweight

Incidence is the measure of the number of events in a given time interval. The incidence of taking the U.S. census is once per decade. Incidence is an important measure in health outcomes, but nothing is simple. For example, the incidence of a serious motor-vehicle accident is much, much greater at speeds between 30 and 50 mph than at faster or slower speeds. All of us would wonder about an inference drawn from these data that proclaimed it was safer to drive slower or faster than 30 to 50 mph. Of course, such an assertion is fallacious. Most driving occurs between 30 and 50 mph. If one corrects the incidence data for the preponderance of time we drive between these speeds, the inference is dramatically differ-

TABLE 1

Canadian Data on All-Cause Mortality as a Function of BMI

BMI	Adjusted Relative Risk (95% Confidence Interval)
<18.5	1.89 (1.36–2.64)
18.5 to <20.0	1.23 (0.86–1.76)
20.0 to <22.5	1.18 (0.98–1.44)
22.5 to <25.0	1.00
25.0 to <27.5	0.93 (0.77–1.12)
27.5 to <30.0	0.87 (0.69–1.10)
30.0 to <32.5	1.08 (0.80–1.85)
32.5 to <35.0	0.92 (0.67–1.26)
35 or greater	148 (1.06–2.06)

ent. The likelihood of an accident at speeds over 50 mph is dramatically higher. The amount of time we spend at each speed is a critical measure, a known *confounder* to interpreting the raw incidence data. Whenever we use raw data, even data we think is not so raw, we need to wonder about unknown confounders that may render the obvious interpretation totally wrong. Confounders are one of the Horsemen of the Statistical Apocalypse. Never forget that. The risks of obesity are an object lesson.

Body Mass Index (BMI) is a standard measure of heft that considers both weight and height; it is the weight in kilograms divided by the square of the height in meters. It's not a perfect measure, but it's a reasonable approximation. "Normal" is defined by "consensus" to be between 18.5 and 25. This consensus was reached by a committee of the World Health Organization. BMI of 25–30 is "overweight," BMI of 30–35 is obese, and over 35 is morbidly obese. Morbid obesity is a marker of those who will die before their time, before "normal" folk. Both underweight (BMI < 18.5) and morbid obesity are mortal hazards in all data sets. There is no argument. However, there is an argument as to how dangerous it is to be overweight or even obese. Recently, Canadian epidemiologists published their analysis of the relationship between BMI and longevity.[12] Their data is presented in Table 1.

A representative sample of community-dwelling Canadians aged twenty-five or older in the 1994/1995 National Population Health Survey was followed for over a decade. There were nearly 2,000 deaths among over 11,000 people during this period of observation. In addition to BMI, this cohort could be stratified by sex, age, smoking habits, physical activity, and daily alcohol consumption. There are statistical manipulations that allow one to take all of these sociodemographic factors and health behaviors into account when calculating the relationship between BMI and mortality. That is what is meant by "Adjusted" in Table 1; the analysis attempts to isolate only the relationship of BMI to mortality. A significant increased risk of mortality over the twelve years of follow-up was observed for the underweight (BMI < 18.5; relative risk = 1.73, P < 0.001) and the morbidly obese (BMI > 35; relative risk = 1.36, P < 0.05). "Relative risk" (RR) is essentially a measure of the probability of dying before people with a BMI of 18.5–25. In this study, the underweight are nearly twice as likely (73 percent) to die before people of "normal" heft. Relative risk is a calculation based on probabilities; it itself is a "likeliest" result. The "95 Percent Confidence Interval" is a measure of the range of values the relative risk is likely to lie between. If the range crosses 1.0, then it is unlikely that there is any increased or decreased risk. So only the abnormally thin and the morbidly obese incur any increased risk of death before their time from their heft. Overweight and obese Canadians are normal in that regard.

This result is echoed by a study of similar design from Australia targeting elderly people living in the community.[13] This cohort study started with nearly 10,000 men and women aged seventy to seventy-five in 1996 and followed them for a decade or until death. Nearly 2,500 had died by the end of the observation period. These investigators went to even greater lengths to isolate the effect of BMI on mortality independent of age, gender, marital status, education, tobacco abuse, alcohol exposure, exercise level, and presence of comorbidities (hypertension, diabetes, stroke, or lung or heart disease). Comorbidities are indications of general health status. The risk of death was 13 percent *lower* for overweight elderly people (95 Percent Confidence Interval = 0.78–0.94) than for those of normal weight. The risk of death was indistinguishable for obese and normal-weight people (95 Percent Confidence Interval = 0.85–1.11). Of all the other competing influences, being sedentary doubled the mortality risk for women across all levels of BMI; being sedentary was a mortal hazard for men, too, but not as powerful.

We will have more to say about "lifestyle," such as diet and exercise, below. But for now, let's step back and consider the cognitive dissonance generated by these two studies. After all, we are bombarded with fore-warnings about the implications of the epidemic of obesity. These two studies were published in 2009 and 2010, respectively. Before these ap-peared, there were over fifty prospective studies leading to contrary con-clusions;[14] the mortal risk escalated for any BMI higher than 25 by about 30 percent for every 5 kg/m² of BMI. The problem is that while all these earlier studies "adjusted" their statistics for age, gender, and smoking, they were uneven in adjusting for other sociodemographic variables, for other health behaviors, and for comorbidities. It's back to our example of how ignoring the time of exposure leads to the fallacious inference that you're safer driving faster than 50 mph. One cannot speak about the risk of one attribute — BMI — without considering the influences of all the coincident attributes that might be playing a role. And even then, one can only hope there isn't another that you didn't recognize or couldn't measure. That's why the best you can do is to generate an inference that stands today because it has yet to be refuted. Such is the tentative nature of "truth."

When there are multiple competing influences on a given outcome such as mortality, there is lots of room for debate as to the appropriate statistics to apply. Books are written about this. The analysis of the mor-tality data in the United States is illustrative of all the computational challenges. Through its National Health and Nutrition Examination Sur-vey (NHANES) program, the National Center for Health Statistics of the Centers for Disease Control and Prevention (CDC) has been conducting longitudinal surveys of the health of the general population for genera-tions. The NHANES I cohort was selected and recruited between 1971 and 1973, NHANES II between 1976 and 1980, and NHANES III between 1988 and 1994. All have been followed closely ever since. In 2007 Katherine Flegal and her colleagues published an analysis of the excess deaths and their causes for people who were underweight, overweight, and obese when the cohorts were assembled.[15] The combined study sample was about 37,000, and about one-third had died by 2004. The statistic used determined the relative risk for excess deaths in each category of BMI and took into account sex and race as well as tobacco and alcohol exposure at inception of the cohorts. But there is a problem in combining the three cohorts: they are different in the length of follow-up, and it is likely that the complexion of the "general population" that was sampled had changed between 1970 and 1990. Researchers therefore compared two analyses. In one, the "balanced follow-up," they tried to correct for the differences in

TABLE 2

Excess Deaths as a Percentage of All Deaths (95% Confidence Interval) Based on the Combined NHANES I, II, and III Data Sets

Causes of Death	Underweight (BMI <18.5)	Normal (BMI 18.5 to <25)	Overweight (BMI 25 to <30)	Obese (BMI ≥30)
Balanced Follow-up				
CVD*	1.0 (0.0–2.0)	0 (Reference)	−2.0 (−5.9–1.9)	9.4 (6.0–12.9)
Cancer	0.8 (−0.4–1.9)	0 (Reference)	−2.5 (−8.1–3.1)	2.7 (−2.5–7.9)
Other	3.6 (1.9–5.4)	0 (Reference)	−11.8 (−16.3–7.3)	−0.1 (−4.5–4.4)
Total Followup				
CVD	0.5 (−0.2–1.1)	0 (Reference)	2.4 (−0.7–5.5)	13.1 (10.2–15.9)
Cancer	0.3 (−0.4–1.0)	0 (Reference)	1.2 (−3.3–5.8)	2.8 (−1.4–7.0)
Other	2.6 (1.3–3.8)	0 (Reference)	−7.6 (−11.0–4.1)	3.9 (−0.1–7.9)

*CVD = Cardiovascular causes of death

Source: Table adapted from K. M. Flegal, B. I. Graubard, D. F. Williamson, and M. H. Gail, Cause-specific excess deaths associated with underweight, overweight, and obesity, *Journal of the American Medical Association* 2007; 298: 2028–37.

the cohorts that they could ascribe to length of follow-up; and in the "total follow-up," they made no such correction. The relative risks for excess death for each calculation as a function of BMI is presented in Table 2.

Remember, the 95 Percent Confidence Interval means the actual number will fall somewhere within the limit 95 times out of 100. If the Confidence Limit crosses 1.0, that means the result could be either higher or lower than the reference value—in other words, the particular BMI might either harm or help. You can impute meaning to such a result depending on how much of a gambler you are. If you're not much of a gambler and therefore conform to convention, there is no excess in deaths from being overweight, even if the calculation is based on the total combined cohort with or without balancing for the different lengths of follow-up of each cohort. Contrary to the findings in the Canadian and Australian populations, there appears to be an important risk for excess cardiovascular deaths in the obese American population. Is this a reflection of different approaches to statistical modeling of the data? Is this a reflection of important differences in the complexion of the populations? Or is it both? After all, we know the income gaps and other measures of socioeconomic and psychosocial context differ between these countries, perhaps to a degree that overwhelms the approximations used in the statistical modeling of the data.

The failure to demonstrate any hazard from being overweight caused few waves — initially. That was not the case when subsequent analyses of these data were published in January 2010, again in the prestigious *Journal of the American Medical Association.*[16] They could detect no trends toward increasing BMI after 1999 in American adults or children, except among the very heaviest of boys aged six to nineteen. What? There's no obesity epidemic? These papers provoked a firestorm in the epidemiology, health-policy, and patient-advocacy communities — not to mention all the purveyors of ways to lose weight. The dust settled, particularly after the director of the CDC backpedaled on the inferences and other statisticians pummeled the data so that alternative interpretations were apparent. This episode should not inflame our collective cynicism. Rather, it is an object lesson in the tentative nature of "truth," which is ever more tentative when we look for small effects in large populations and hope that the confounders are silenced.

Is My Lifestyle Better Than Yours?

This brings us to the next set of issues that all in their Golden Years have been told are pressing. In the spirit of disclosure, I am an "aged worker" for whom Golden Years is not an abstraction. Therefore, despite all my efforts and high intentions, I will bring my personal perspective and my projections to bear on the primitive, inconclusive science that informs the answer to the query that introduces this section. That is how it always is, and always will be, when science is no match or barely a match for a critical question. I will attempt to fess up as we go along.

There is a crucial distinction between the health of the person and the health of the people. The health of any person is a composite of the degree to which one feels invincible or at least in control, the preconceptions one has as to biological prerequisites for doing well going forward, and the feedback one gets from one's community. The health of the people is an epidemiologic construct viewed in the light of communitarian ethics.

I have no reason to question your approach to your own health. I don't care if you feel kale is better for you than cookie-dough ice cream. I don't care if you are a vegan or a zealot for anything with olive oil. I don't care if you avoid meat or avoid fish. I don't care if you feel better for having ingested a potpourri of supplements. I don't care if you stretch, or medi-tate, or jog, or choose to have your colon irrigated. I don't care—with two caveats.

First, there must be assurance that you are doing yourself no harm. Much of the stuff marketed as promoting "wellness" has impurities, some interacts with prescription medicines to cause harm, and some is poten-tially harmful itself. If you're going to be a consumer, be an informed con-sumer. Memorial Sloan-Kettering Cancer Center has a website discussing herbal supplements.[17] The FDA considers the safety and purity of supple-ments a priority; the FDA's website is a portal to the state of this science.[18]

Second, you should be fully informed that participation in *any* pro-gram, regimen, or other intervention purporting to enhance your health will change you forever—even if you are disappointed by the outcome. You will learn new idioms, new body images, and new expectations. And you will join a new peer group testing the same waters if not already im-mersing themselves in them. If you've fractured your arm, you have little choice but to enter the world of orthopedics and rehabilitation. Before choosing to undergo cancer chemotherapy, you should demand sufficient explanation as to the benefits and risks so that the choice is informed, because entering into treatment is as life altering as the cancer itself. The best you can hope for is to spend the rest of your life as a "survivor." That makes sense if you were really benefited. We will discuss the notion of "cure" in the context of prostate or breast cancer in the next chapter and will return to it with vigor in chapter 7. For many diseases like cancer, there is an extensive scientific literature that can inform decision making. But for much of the menu purporting to enhance your health, there is no informative science. Before you choose from that menu, you should care-fully consider its perceptual ramifications. Do you want to join the cadre of people who need this particular option to feel well?

Of course, if you so choose, and it's safe, and it makes you feel good even though it's untested or unsubstantiated by scientific testing or sim-ply a sectarian belief in the realm of metaphysics, who am I to criticize? However, I do have a problem with being asked to share the expense in the underwriting of what amount to unfounded, personal health convic-tions. And beware the guru, the true believer, and other features of sectar-ian health purveyance. This has a colorful but often reprehensible history. Don't be taken in.

Harsh? Infuriating? I don't expect you to let me off easily with my highfalutin reliance on the available science. Science is seldom, if ever, a match for "lifestyle" hypothesis testing. Lifestyle is not one-dimensional; it's not a pill we may or may not take. It is highly variable in its details over time for any one of us. Furthermore, humanity is a sea of individual differences, thankfully. No two of us are the same; that's why we need poets. How many vegans were sedentary for decades before deciding to transition to athletic carnivores? Who among us can really quantify what they were doing or eating last year, let alone last month? How many years must we observe any person or group before we are convinced we have observed long enough to declare the observation a valid glimpse of their lifestyle? How closely must we observe, or can we simply rely on recall? And how much of our fate is determined early on in life, even heritable? Studying "lifestyle" systematically requires a tremendous amount of self-confidence — or is it bravado or hubris, and an equal amount of skepticism?

Exercise

Exercise is more than musculoskeletal functioning; it's *optional* musculoskeletal functioning. As a student of workplace health and safety, I have long been amused by America's zeal for exercise promulgated in glossy magazines, by talking heads on television, by presidential commissions, and the like. But it is always promulgated by people who are wont to wear specialized garments to undertake the physical exertion they consider good for their health. Their advice and pronouncements falls most readily on the ears of those of like mind and proclivity. However, there are many people for whom a different context applies. For example, if you are tired and sweaty at the end of eight hours of loading trucks or stacking boxes in a warehouse at wages not far from minimum, wouldn't you find advice to walk up stairs instead of taking an elevator ludicrous? How about if you were a professional gardener, or spent the day harvesting tobacco or strawberries? Jogging on the road, an hour of step aerobics, or an hour on a cross trainer in a gymnasium might also engender cognitive dissonance. There are many people whose employment is physically demanding, including many for whom the toiling is aerobic. We don't call that "exercise," do we? And, as we've discussed, these folks who toil for low wages are less likely to enjoy Golden Years than those who have the means and the leisure time to work out in Lycra.

Why are we so fixated on "exercise" as a national "health" agenda? Certainly, it promulgates an enormous industry that services this agenda with clubs, garments, gadgets, machines, and whatever. But does it promulgate "health"? The reflexive answer is the circular reasoning that we have an "obesity" epidemic because we are a nation of couch potatoes. If we "exercise," will we lose weight? Possibly, but it's a daunting undertaking. If you push yourself hard for an hour of aerobic exercise, you can allow yourself one glazed donut. Elite athletes in endurance sports must pay attention to caloric intake to compensate for expenditure. Recreational athletes have no such challenge. If you want to lose weight, consume less food.

There's another diabolical truth about caloric expenditure: thinking, even thinking great thoughts, is exceedingly efficient from a metabolic standpoint. The countless hours I have spent writing this book consumed the equivalent of a glazed donut or two. Truth be told, I have been a recreational cyclist for decades. I ride more than 100 miles per week, almost always the same hilly thirty-mile loop at about 16 mph. It is my custom to cycle alone, enjoying the beauty of the countryside while rethinking whatever I've been writing at the time. I can tell you how many miles each chapter required. So this book has caused me to enjoy many an hour at peace with the world and allowed me to consume more than one glazed donut equivalent without adding to my already substantial padding. I have no idea what I weigh because I never weigh myself, but I can't fool myself into thinking I've lost even an ounce.

Exercise can be advocated in the service of vanity. Both the fact of exercising and the degree to which one's skin is taut are badges of "wellness" and cause for strutting, particularly in the Lycra crowd. Society at the turn of this century holds thinness up for envy to the same degree that society at the turn of the last century considered thinness a sign of social deprivation. One of the contributions of the Women's Health Study is to document the effort that must be expended in the quest of this element of vanity.[19] From 1992 to 2004, the Women's Health Study randomized nearly 40,000 well women to test if low-dose aspirin and vitamin E prevented heart disease and cancer. At the end of the study, 34,000 of the women who were still well agreed to continue in an observational study. Only women who had a BMI under 25 at the inception of the study were able to avoid weight gain over time, and only *if* they exercised seriously about sixty minutes a day.

If exercise has so little effect on BMI, what "health" benefit is being touted as the national agenda? Do you live longer for being fit? Or do you live longer because you have the time, inclination, and wherewithal to stay in shape? The argument for the former stems from a study conducted by the Cooper Institute for Aerobics Research of the fate of "well-educated" men and women who attended the Cooper Clinic between 1970 and 1989. Some 25,000 men and 7,000 women who had traveled to Houston to participate in the wellness program formulated by Kenneth Cooper of "aerobics" fame were followed for an average of eight years, during which time very few had died: 601 men and 89 women.[20] Lots of clinical information was gathered when these people enrolled in the program, including their aerobic capacity; all study participants achieved at least 85 percent of their age-predicted heart rate running on a treadmill, though the less fit took longer to get there. There were very few obese people in this study. The few who died during the follow-up tended to do less well on the treadmill at baseline. The Cooper Institute argues, therefore, that aerobic fitness is life prolonging. This interpretation downplays that the less fit were also a bit older, more likely to have abused tobacco, and more likely to consider themselves less "healthy" at baseline.

There is a lot more scientific literature desperately trying to document longevity-promoting benefits of exercise. The science supporting the hypothesis is tenuous. The conviction that exercise is beneficial is anything but tentative. In 2008 the U.S. government issued a guideline that recommends at least 150 minutes a week of moderate-intensity aerobic physical activity for individuals to obtain "substantial health benefits."[21] The membership of the committee formulating these guidelines was comprised of many for whom the benefits of exercise were the focus of their investigative and clinical careers. They were so prone to be swayed by the plethora of very small benefits that they were comfortable emphasizing the relative reductions in adverse outcomes rather than the absolute reductions. I was pretty dismissive of the results of the Cooper Institute study. I doubt you would be as dismissive if I told you there was a 50 percent increased risk of death if you were an unfit man and a 100 percent increased risk if you were an unfit woman. I didn't state this, although it is true, because the absolute death rates are hardly as dramatic. If you follow 10,000 "highly educated" but "unfit" men for a year, 46 would die; but if you follow 10,000 "fit" men for a year, only 30 would die. For women, the absolute death rates would be 30/10,000 women/year and 15/10,000 women/year, respectively. In other words, if you get 1,000 people to exercise for a year, you may spare one or two of them death before their time. That's a lot of fitness advocacy for a gain that is so small that one wonders what confounder is lurking that might better explain it, or even if it is reproducible.

The Cooper Institute study discussed above is an observational cohort study; they defined the fitness of the subjects at baseline and determined their fate by following them over time. Such a study is considered hypothesis generating at best. If it has greater value, it is to the extent that it fails to discern associations between exposure (fitness as a "surrogate measure," or representation of exercise) and health effect (survival). To test the hypothesis requires a different experimental design, one that tries to control for all the known confounders and randomizes the population hoping to equalize the unmeasured confounders. To their credit, the Cooper Institute was the setting for such a randomized controlled trial.[22] They randomized nearly 500 sedentary, postmenopausal, overweight or obese women to one of four groups. One group carried on in their previous fashion; the others participated in exercise groups that met three to four times per week for six months and were designed to achieve either one-half of the public-health weekly recommended exercise level, the full level, or 50 percent more. Guess what? The more they exercised, the more fit they became as measured by their metabolic efficiency. There was no change in blood pressure, blood lipids, or blood glucose, and the study was too brief to expect any change in survival or disease outcomes by exercising three hours per week. But if you believe there will be, or believe there will be if you exercise even more vigorously, then you're in accord with the author of the editorial that accompanied this paper. I remain a skeptic.

Nonetheless, I am going to strongly urge all who are of Golden Age to stay fit if they already are fit and to get fit if they're not. This is not a projection growing out of my joy in cycling or my own vanity. Rather, for all of us, chapter 5, figuratively and literally, is looming: nearly all of us will acquire a degree of decrepitude. It may be a minor degree, and it may come late in our lifeline. But don't gamble. You are much better off postponing decrepitude or diminishing its intensity than trying to recover function once it has set in. It is relatively easy to show that exercise can improve balance and diminish falls in elderly people, at least in the short term.[23] It is also easy to show that exercise can prevent and treat osteopenia (diminished bone calcium) in postmenopausal women, although it is not clear that this translates into fewer fractures,[24] as we'll discuss in chapter 5.

But I have a far more practical reason for urging those in their Golden Years to get fit and/or stay fit. The slide toward decrepitude is gradual, though its slope differs from person to person. Many activities of daily living that you take for granted now will prove more challenging before long. Getting off the floor may not be pretty now, but it may not be possible then. Rising from a seated position, let alone a squat, can be daunting. Reaching for a thirty-pound parcel several feet away is a physically demanding task now, and it may be prohibitive then. I'm not just envisioning your golf game or the next trip to the market. Try playing with a toddler. Your Golden Years will stay golden longer if you can obviate some of the biomechanical compromises that accompany decrepitude.

Easier said than done? It's less of a challenge if you have a lifelong proclivity for fitness activities. If you don't, I could prescribe such, though the effectiveness of such a prescription merits consideration. There have been very few studies of the results of a medically prescribed exercise program for community residents. One was undertaken in Wellington, New Zealand.[25] After baseline evaluation, relatively inactive women were randomized to usual care or to receive a brief nurse-led discussion of physical activity followed by monthly telephone support and a six-month follow-up visit. The intervention group reported an impressive increase in exercise intensity and in mental-health scores. But the only noteworthy change in clinical outcomes was that those in the exercise intervention group incurred *more* falls and slightly more injuries. There is a similar ongoing trial in Britain with well elderly people in the community looking at alternative exercise regimens.[26] Time will tell in this elderly population, although it is discouraging that no clinical benefit was discerned in another study in which subjects were recruited because of a family history of diabetes.[27]

Maybe one's personal preferences in lifestyle are too entrenched to be undone by my prescription. Maybe the best I can do is to cajole and forewarn. Seldom do I learn that someone has taken up a fitness regimen for the first time in the privacy of his or her home. I have many patients who have tucked an exercise bicycle into a closet, where it is accumulating dust. There is far more success if the activity involves a peer group and is not medicalized. Furthermore, there is far more success both in initiation and in persistence if the exercise is appealing and "forgiving." As for "forgiving" exercises, riding an exercise bicycle and using a stair climber are less likely to be thwarted by the intermittent regional musculoskeletal disorders (backache, knee pain, etc.) that are common at all ages and more persistent as we age. Participating in water aerobics programs can be all things to most people.

Enough said. You get the idea.

Diet

For similar reasons, I am going to urge all in their Golden Years who are flirting with obesity to not to cross the line and those who are obese to take this opportunity to move toward just being overweight. As we've discussed, this advice is not in the service of longevity (except for those who are morbidly obese and who are already in trouble.) Heft challenges our biomechanics. If you're moving quickly, you put several times your body weight across weight-bearing joints with each heel strike. The converse is the good news; for every ten pounds you lose, you ask thirty to fifty pounds less of your knees with each heel strike and spare your bunions nearly as much during push off. When it comes to biomechanics, non-weight-bearing exercise and weight loss provide prompt gratification when weight-bearing joints are symptomatic.

And, as we've discussed, if you want to lose weight, cut back on your caloric intake. As long as you're not unreasonable, I don't care what you eat to accomplish the reduction in caloric intake. There have been many small, short-term studies, all with design flaws, purporting benefit for one macronutrient or another. None are convincing, let alone compelling. Of the few that had extended for at least a year, several could not show the superiority of diets that were either high or low in carbohydrates, protein, or fat; the "CALERIE" trial and a National Institutes of Health–supported two-year trial are representative examples.[28] Other studies found that a vegetarian diet that is very high in carbohydrates and very low in fat beats a standard low-fat diet,[29] or that a low-carbohydrate, Mediterranean-style diet was associated with more weight loss than a low-fat diet.[30] Many more studies contributed to the cacophony of those who were advocating, if not hawking, their weight-loss diet. As far as I was concerned, Atkins's high-fat, low carbohydrate advocacy and Pritikin's converse could be shelved in the historical archives next to many predecessors while leaving shelf space for all the successors.

The trial published by Frank Sacks and his colleagues in the *New England Journal of Medicine* in 2009 places substantial scientific grounding under my assertion.[31] Over 800 obese adults were randomized to one of four diets: high fat with either average or high protein or low fat with either average or high protein. The carbohydrate content varied from 35 to 65 percent, so that the caloric intake of each individual represented a deficit of 750 kcal per day from their baseline energy expenditure. Group sessions with behavioral counseling were held nearly weekly for the first six months and biweekly for the remainder of the two-year trial. The goal for moderate exercise was ninety minutes per week. Neither the participants nor the staff were aware of the diet anyone consumed, since all had similar foods. Regardless of the diet, everyone lost about 6 percent of weight and of waist circumference at six months and then drifted back toward their baseline over the subsequent 18 months. All diets improved risk factors for cardiovascular disease and diabetes. There were differences, but these were predictable consequences of the complexion of the diet.

Also, there is no compelling prospective data to support the public-health mantra that dietary saturated fat is associated with an increased risk of cardiovascular disease. There is a cacophony similar to the weight-loss diet claims, but in a recent attempt to make sense of the long-term studies, little hazard from dietary saturated fats was discerned.[32] I should point out that while this analysis was undertaken by a premier endocrinologist, Ronald M. Krauss and his colleagues, their efforts were supported by the National Institutes of Health *and* the National Dairy Council. Suffice it to say that the hazardous nature of dietary saturated fat is yet another hypothesis that has taken on a life of its own despite the inability of science to provide firm underpinning, but not for lack of trying.

Decreasing caloric intake need not require a dramatic change in dietary habits. Cut back on your average caloric intake by 10 percent and you will be rewarded with a gradual weight loss that is less susceptible to recidivism — that is, yo-yo weight loss. The secret is in knowing where in your daily intake to find the most pain-free and dispensable equivalent of a glazed donut or two. There are books about this and dieticians and nutritionists to regale you. There's also some common sense and relevant information hiding on many labels. Beware of sweetened beverages and sweetened foods, beware of breads and pastas, beware of fried foods, and be aware. Out of sight helps with out of mind. And stay away from the remaining licensed prescription pharmaceuticals that are marketed as shortcuts to weight loss. Their effectiveness is modest at best and less consistent then their specific adverse effects.[33]

The Risk-Factor Fetish

As I said before, Americans know their numbers. Americans know their cholesterol, even their HDL and LDL cholesterol. They know their blood pressure. Many know their blood sugar and more and more their hemoglobin-A1c (HbA1c), the test that measures blood sugar over time. Since the normal cutoff for all of these is defined at the last meeting of some committee, usually dominated by members of the relevant medical specialty, "normal" is a moving target. At the rate these committees are going, fewer and fewer of us will qualify as "normal" until we're down to the "Last Well Person" in the title of my 2004 book. Speaking of my books, in *Worried Sick* (2008) I discuss the "risk factor" concept in great detail. Rather than reproduce that discussion here, I will provide three more recent object lessons on the flawed reasoning and hidden agendas that keep "risk factors" in the headlines and on our minds. These are lessons that will make you a match for pharmaceutical marketing and arm you to participate in medical decision making for the rest of your life.

Crestor® by Jove

On March 31, 2008, the pharmaceutical giant AstraZeneca trumpeted the early stopping of the JUPITER trial. After only two years, there was "unequivocal evidence" that AstraZeneca's cholesterol-lowering statin drug, Rosuvastatin (Crestor), was too effective to withhold it from anyone who was well and had normal cholesterol levels but had an elevation in another normal blood constituent, the high-sensitivity C-reactive protein (hsCRP). For reasons I detail in *Worried Sick* and have discussed widely, including in the *Washington Post*, I am unwilling to let anyone test my cholesterol. Not only is it a weak risk factor in well people, but there is also no compelling evidence that even if my cholesterol was "high," swallowing any statin would benefit me. Certainly, taking a statin would not spare me from a fatal heart attack or stroke. The data that it would spare me from a nonfatal heart attack is tenuous. I won't let anyone check my cholesterol until I see unequivocal data that taking a statin yields meaningful benefit for me. Now, regardless of my cholesterol level, AstraZeneca wants me to get my hsCRP measured so that I can swallow Crestor if it's elevated. Eleven months after the pronouncement of success, during which the sales of Crestor and market value of AstraZeneca flourished, the results of JUPITER were published in the online edition of the *New England Journal Medicine*.[34] Paul Ridker of the Brigham and Women's Hospital in Boston was the first author and lead investigator. I lambasted the publication the day it was published.[35] There are many devils in its details.

AstraZeneca and Ridker are preaching to the risk-factor choir. It is the dream of all physicians and of the science of public health that we would someday be able to predict illness and intervene successfully while the person is well. Polio and smallpox vaccination schemes were not targeted at individuals but served the health of the public in this fashion. If the intervention is less effective, then one has to weigh its likelihood for adverse effects and its cost. The formulation that holds sway to this day was put forth many years ago by Geoffrey Rose in Britain.[36] If there is an imperfect medical intervention, it should be reserved for those at greatest risk for the disease. The "low-risk" population should be spared medical interventions and offered more general advice, even though the low-risk population will have a greater burden of disease by virtue of being much larger than the "high-risk" subset. Hence, we are urged to prescribe statins for those at high risk and advise "diet" for the masses.

When it comes to cardiovascular disease and other diseases of later life, profiling risk is challenging, given the time it takes to witness the outcome. People who have already had a heart attack are "high risk" for another heart attack. For this group, while the benefit of statin therapy is far from impressive, it is generally accepted that statin therapy is indicated. This is termed "secondary prevention." But we are concerned in this chapter with "primary prevention," prevention for people who have not suffered a heart attack. In order to profile risk for primary prevention, epidemiology is invested in "surrogate measures," tests that may not measure a disease itself but should speak to the chances of developing the disease.

Cholesterol is such a surrogate measure. If you have high cholesterol, you will not know it unless I tell you, and most people will be no worse off for it. "High risk" is a statistical calculation, not a clinical test; if you fall into the worst LDL/HDL category in the Framingham stratification, you are at *risk* of dying a year or two sooner than those in the low-risk categories. For most that are labeled "high risk," the risk is small, and estimates by extrapolation are of the order of months—for which you are prescribed a lifetime of statin swallowing. Given that it is not clear that lowering the cholesterol leads to a meaningful reduction in risk, I am not alone in decrying the use of statins for the primary prevention of cardiovascular disease.[37]

AstraZeneca and Ridker are not dissuaded. They are assiduously trying to tease more "high-risk" folks out of the "low-risk" stratum. AstraZeneca and Ridker are somewhat attached at the hip: Ridker holds the patent on the high-sensitivity CRP assay with his Boston hospital, Brigham and Women's, and is a paid consultant and grant recipient from AstraZeneca and other pharmaceutical firms. In the best of worlds, it is difficult to avoid unscientific influences when pharmaceutical firms contract research to academic organizations—and JUPITER is ripe with potential conflicts of interest.[38]

The JUPITER trial cost AstraZeneca a great deal of money, largely to compensate the participating physicians and their institutions. It is a Herculean drug trial designed not solely to demonstrate a change in a surrogate outcome (cholesterol levels) but to see if Crestor decreases the incidence of untoward clinical events. Physicians in over 1,300 centers in twenty-six countries contracted to recruit subjects. They screened some 90,000 people and enrolled nearly 18,000 well people with elevated hsCRPs but normal blood lipids. At each center, half the recruits were randomly assigned to swallow a placebo pill, the other half Crestor. The intent was to monitor this army of volunteers for five years to see if the groups differed in their incidence of any of the following: heart attack, stroke, hospitalization for unstable angina or for surgery on their coronary arteries, and death from cardiovascular causes. Such clustering of multiple, often disparate clinical events into a single "composite outcome" measure is common practice in cardiovascular (and oncology) drug trials.

JUPITER, as is true for all modern trials, had an oversight committee charged with breaking the code periodically to see if the volunteers on Crestor were fairing better or worse than the volunteers on placebo. The JUPITER oversight committee is comprised of luminaries in the world of cardiology who, like nearly all the principal JUPITER trial investigators, had declared financial involvements with the industry that serves the cardiovascular enterprise, many with AstraZeneca. After 1.9 years, the oversight committee sounded the alarm when they noted a highly statistically significant reduction in the incidence of the feared outcomes—a reduction of 56 percent. That number was placed up front in the abstract of the paper and in the media; 56 percent reduction is hard to ignore. One imagines that if you put two of four people on Crestor, two years later, both on Crestor would be alive but only one of the other pair would be. If that were true, I'd have my hsCRP tested today. But that's not even close to the truth.

At the end of two years, about 2 percent of the 18,000 subjects had suffered any of the cardiovascular outcomes. Of those on Crestor, 1.6 percent were stricken, while 2.8 percent of those not afforded Crestor were—a difference of 1.2 percent. However, not all of these people were in the trial for all of the first two years; they entered at different times, reflecting the vagaries of recruitment. A more accurate reflection that takes this into account is to calculate for every 100 how many would have suffered one of the cardiovascular outcomes in a year in the trial. This event rate for any of the events in the "composite outcome" is 0.77 on Crestor and 1.36 without Crestor. That's the 56 percent reduction that is being trumpeted. That means I'd have to treat about 200 well people with Crestor for a year to spare one any of these cardiovascular events. But the four cardiac outcomes were not equally represented. I'd have to treat about 400 well people for a year to spare one a nonfatal heart attack, about 600 to spare one a stroke. I am unwilling to even suggest a life-saving benefit.

So the relative reduction of 56 percent turns out to be an absolute reduction of 0.59 percent. If you don't want to dismiss this as much ado about nothing out of hand, at least pause and reflect before you swallow Crestor or before my colleagues prescribe it. Consider these questions:

Are you convinced this small effect is real and that it will reproduce if one were to repeat the JUPITER *trial?* I am not. I am reflexively skeptical of effects of this magnitude. My main reason relates to the nature of the randomized controlled trials we rely on for evidence. There are many factors vying to seal a well person's cardiovascular fate. For example, there are other so-called cardiovascular risk factors, such as obesity and tobacco abuse. By assigning volunteers randomly to Crestor or placebo, one hopes that the number of smokers and obese folks are equal in the two groups. When the JUPITER investigators checked, indeed such measurable risk factors were distributed 50:50. One has to have faith that the factors that cannot be safely measured (such as the degree to which the blood vessels are diseased) also distribute 50:50. And one has to have faith that the factors that JUPITER was designed to ignore distribute 50:50 as well. Socioeconomic status, job security, and education level are even more important risk factors that are independent of those measured and likely to vary widely across the research sites in these twenty-six countries. Slight imbalances between the Crestor and placebo groups could result in effects of the magnitude touted by JUPITER. I never leap to act on the basis of such small effects. They're why if you feed your family margarine tonight at dinner, you're not a caring person, while last year it was butter that was bad for you. However, Ridker and Robert Glynn, the study statistician, are convinced that if they screened all adults in America with normal blood-cholesterol levels and treated those with an elevated hsCRP with Crestor, they could spare some 250,000 Americans the composite outcome each year.

Do you think it was appropriate to have stopped the trial early? Certainly, if there's a dramatic incidence of adverse effects, a trial should be stopped. Possibly, if there's a dramatic incidence of major, unequivocal positive effects, one could argue for stopping early But this is a tenuous argument even for large positive effects and untenable for small effects.[39] Small effects come and go, and sometimes they even reverse polarity during the prolonged course of a trial such as JUPITER. Surveillance for small benefits predisposes to detecting a nondurable wobble.

If you're convinced these small effects are real, are they meaningful to you? Are you willing to swallow Crestor every day for two years in the hopes that you're the one in hundreds who just might be spared one of the outcomes in the composite? Does it bother you that more of the volunteers on Crestor were diagnosed with diabetes? Aside from diabetes, the volunteers for JUPITER were not harmed in the two years. But that does not mean the drug is risk free. Does it bother you that the occasional person on Crestor dies from muscle disease caused by Crestor, and some have liver or kidney irritation? In the first five years since it was licensed, Crestor caused over 100 cases of destructive muscle disease (rhabdomyolysis)—not as often as another statin, Baycol, which was withdrawn from the market, but not trivial. I am not tormented by such risks, as I doubt the small benefits are real and therefore have no interest in taking or prescribing Crestor. You and your prescribing physician should take pause, at the very least. Realize that survey data from Britain suggest that if you treat about 35 people with any statin for five years, you increase the risk of cataract for one of them. The comparable "Number Needed to Harm" (NNH) for kidney failure is 400, 250 for moderate-to-severe muscle trouble, and 150 for moderate-to-severe liver trouble.[40]

Do you believe that hsCRP is a meaningful risk factor? This is Ridker's contention. He bases it largely on adding the measurement of hsCRP to a randomized placebo-controlled trial of lovastatin (another statin) that was published a decade ago.[41] The absolute difference in composite cardiovascular outcome between subjects on placebo with low LDL cholesterol who had a high hsCRP and those with a low hsCRP was about 1.5 percent with eight years of follow-up. In other words, about 99.5 percent of subjects with low hsCRP were spared any of the events in the composite outcome, as compared to 98 percent of subjects with a high hsCRP. But even this tiny difference in risk is open to question. The measurement of hsCRP is difficult both methodologically and because it normally wobbles around one's set point. Furthermore, CRP levels are genetically controlled, and the genes have nothing to do with the risk of cardiovascular disease.[42] Maybe the known associations of hsCRP level with BMI, gender, age, minor inflammatory stimuli (such as cigarette smoke and air pollutants), or estrogen-containing medicines would explain the small differences Ridker is trumpeting.[43]

And trumpeting he is. JUPITER leaves a mountain of data in its wake that is begging to be mined. True, one needs a statistical canary to return to the mine repeatedly; in fact, most of us feel it shouldn't be done. Before doing a trial, one establishes a primary hypothesis to be tested and maybe a secondary hypothesis. But if you mine the data repeatedly, you're likely to come up with fool's gold. Let's say there's really no difference between subjects treated with Crestor and any outcome. If you probe for 100 different outcomes, you're likely to be fooled five times. Intrepid Ridker is mining these data repeatedly to see if Crestor improves peripheral arterial disease, or thromboembolic (blood clots from veins) disease, or . . .

Ridker and his colleagues were even willing to pick at the JUPITER data in an "exploratory analysis," from which they conclude that rosuvastatin might be useful in primary prevention of heart disease in people over 70 with an elevated hsCRP, a conclusion applauded in an accompanying editorial.[44] An "exploratory analysis" is never more than hypothesis generating. It is the exercise of seeking associations after the data are generated and choosing those that seem worthy of pursuit in a rigorous new study. I wonder how many readers realize the tenuous nature of an "exploratory analysis."

These are my serious academic compunctions. I have even more serious compunctions as a consumer and a citizen. The Crestor and hsCRP and JUPITER rumblings have inserted themselves into the public conscience to an extent that is far more impressive than the underlying science supports. As far as I'm concerned, the science should have sounded the death knell for Ridker's hsCRP-related hypotheses. This story is an excellent example of what Alastair Matheson terms the husbandry of scientific and medical knowledge by the pharmaceutical industry and what others term "spin."[45] Research and marketing activities coalesce around "product canons" that subjugate scientific results to commercial positioning. News media are enablers by frequently failing to report on medications studies accurately, ignoring the corporate sponsorship of drug trials, and often referring to the drugs by brand rather than generic name.[46] Perhaps the most egregious example of this is corporate underwriting of "seed trials," which have the appearance of science but the intent of turning the physicians who participate into "thought leaders" who drive prescribing.[47] This entire corporate husbandry commandeers our conception of risk. Cognitive psychology holds that we conceptualize risk both by analysis and by intuition.[48] The latter is highly experiential and infused with "doses of feeling." The corporate husbandry plays on the intuitive sense of risk and benefit, rendering it far less rational. The result is that we are all too open to the scare of the week and the miracle of the month without the reflexive skepticism we'd bring to bear on the promotions of a used-car salesmen. We are comfortable to be awash in direct-to-consumer marketing that claims to "lower your (surrogate)," "results in an X percent decrease in (relative reduction)," or "helps you with (composite outcome)." The saddest aspect of this sad state of health appreciation is it need not be so. It is easy to present pharmaceutical data in simple tables so that risk taking reverts to the rational.[49] We should demand at least that much.

Rosiglitazone's RECORD

In 2008 the U.S. Preventive Services Task Force (USPSTF)[50] revisited the literature on screening for type 2 diabetes and came up with the same recommendations that they did in 2005. They felt there was some rationale for screening for type 2 diabetes in patients with hypertension. But they could generate no substantive reason to screen in any other asymptomatic adults. The reason for screening hypertensive patients is a suggestion in the literature that the hypertension in patients with type 2 diabetes is more dangerous and more responsive to antihypertensive therapy; it's not to treat the diabetes.

The reason they do not recommend screening nonhypertensive people is the "benefits of tight glycemic control on microvascular clinical outcomes, such as severe visual impairment or end-stage renal disease, take years to become apparent. There is inadequate evidence that early diabetes control as a result of screening provides an incremental benefit for microvascular clinical outcomes compared with initiating treatment after clinical diagnosis. There is inadequate evidence that tight glycemic control significantly reduces macrovascular complications, such as myocardial infarction and stroke."

In other words, there is no evidence that treating type 2 diabetes to lower the blood sugar protects the patient from the feared diseases associated with type 2 diabetes. Better stated, there have been several randomized controlled trials of pharmaceutical treatment compared to usual care, such as advice about dieting and exercise. The patients were as likely to suffer important "macrovascular" disease with or without the drugs. "Macrovascular disease" is accelerated atherosclerosis of larger vessels leading to heart attacks, strokes, insufficient blood flow to the legs resulting in ulcers and amputations, and kidney failure. I review this literature in detail in *Worried Sick*. There is a hint that "microvascular disease" is prevented, but barely a hint. Patients are generally unaware of their "microvascular disease"; it takes a long time for these subtle changes in the retina and kidney function to impair vision or cause renal failure, too long to be meaningful for nearly all patients labeled as type 2 diabetes.

Type 2 diabetes is a biochemical diagnosis. It denotes a sluggish response to dietary sugar ingestion. When we eat and digest a reasonable meal, nutrients, including sugar (glucose), enter the bloodstream. Blood glucose abruptly rises above the fasting value. In response, our pancreas is stimulated to secrete insulin, which allows glucose to enter the cells to be nurtured by this crucial energy source. In the "normal" person, blood glucose returns to the "normal" fasting level within two hours. In some people, the blood glucose takes longer to return to the fasting level, which is usually higher than normal. This usually reflects the insensitivity of the cells to insulin. Such people are defined as having type 2 diabetes. Type 2 diabetes denotes a population at greater risk for the same complications that afflict patients with type 1 diabetes, where insulin itself is missing: damage to large and small blood vessels throughout their body, damage to eyes and kidneys, and death before their time. However, nearly all patients with type 1 diabetes suffer the onset of their disease when they are young, and all must submit to insulin therapy by injection or they will die. People acquire the biology we label type 2 diabetes much later in life, and the associated consequences later yet. Type 2 diabetes can also be treated with insulin, but it is not mandatory. Patients with classic type 2 diabetes do not lack insulin and therefore do not face death on that basis; to the contrary, they are relatively resistant to their own insulin and tend to produce more to compensate. For them, the nuisance and cost of injecting insulin to overcome *insulin resistance* has to be weighed against the uncertain potential for benefit in the long run. That's a hard sell.

Oral hypoglycemic agents are not such a hard sell. They were introduced into the practice of medicine in the 1950s. The "first generation" agents worked mainly by sensitizing the pancreas to secrete more insulin after meals. It made sense that by normalizing glucose metabolism, the risks of type 2 diabetes would be mollified. But sense did not hold up to scientific testing. In one of the pioneering multicenter randomized controlled trials, the "University Group Diabetes Program" (UGDP) set out to study the benefits that accrued from a first-generation oral hypoglycemic compared to diet or insulin therapy.[51] The 1970s were still the early days of doing randomized controlled trials, and as a result, this UGDP trial suffers from some methodological issues that were not fully appreciated at the time. But those issues do not take away from the observation that the patients treated with the first-generation oral hypoglycemic did worse than those in the other two groups, including more deaths. I was early in my career when the results of the UGDP trial were published. I never again prescribed any oral hypoglycemic and vowed I wouldn't until there was data that these agents were beneficial to my patients, not just effective in normalizing their glucose metabolism.

I am still waiting, despite several subsequent generations of oral hypoglycemics. Normalizing the blood sugar of patients labeled as having type 2 diabetes is a mantra of the diabetologists and an enormous profit center for the pharmaceutical industry. After all, by 2004, 21 percent of adults over age sixty qualified for the label, and 1.5 million additional cases are diagnosed each year, according to such agencies as the Agency for Healthcare Research and Quality (AHRQ) of the Center for Medicare Services and the National Diabetes Surveillance System of the CDC. There is an enormous network of basic and clinical investigators who are hell-bent to normalize glucose metabolism. You can find them in the private sector, in universities, and in government facilities. They populate the various committees that define and redefine the limits of normal glucose metabolism and declare and redeclare the appropriate treatment of the abnormality du jour. There is also an enormous financial investment in the type 2 diabetes enterprise — not surprising, given the specter of chronic disease that this "epidemic" represents, not to mention the market for pharmaceutical firms and their fellow travelers. According to the AHRQ News and Numbers (issue no. 288, July 25, 2009), purchases of cholesterol and diabetes prescription drugs by elderly Medicare beneficiaries reached nearly $19 billion in 2007 — approximately one-fourth of the $82 billion spent for medications for the elderly.

The past fifty years of inventiveness has resulted in multiple "me too" new drugs in each successive new class of oral hypoglycemic. Those that have been licensed have in common some impressive ability to normalize glucose metabolism. Some improve other risk factors, such as lipids and BMI, but most are setbacks in that regard. Some have been shown to improve subtle indications of impending damage. But none has been shown to make a clinically meaningful difference in improving longevity, decreasing the incidence of major damage to blood vessels (stroke, heart attack, loss of a limb), or decreasing the incidence of kidney failure or blindness. These disappointments did not stem the tide of treating insulin resistance with pharmaceuticals. Drugs were used in combination and in ever higher doses, even to the point of lowering the blood sugar too far to hypoglycemia, with its risk of dementia in older patients.[52]

Public-health authorities have long been sounding the alarm about type 2 diabetes as yet another epidemic that is ravaging America. In 2006 New York City went so far as to mandate the reporting of blood sugars to monitor the adequacy of treatment of type 2 diabetes because, as Thomas Frieden, the city's health commissioner at the time, said, "We have to get a better handle on what is really the only major health problem in the United States that is getting worse, and getting worse rapidly."[53] "Insulin resistance" was no longer a risk factor; it had become the disease. And an elevated blood sugar, or HbA1c, was no longer a laboratory finding; it was a marker of impending catastrophe, a surrogate for impending stroke or heart attacks or worse. There was a science that should have put this belief system under scrutiny, if not into perspective.[54] For example, a person with diabetes who has yet to have a heart attack is half as likely to have one as the person without diabetes who has already had his or her first. And the persistence in prescribing oral hypoglycemics despite their disappointing efficacy is hard to justify when small changes in lifestyle, such as even a little attention to diet and exercise,[55] does as well. There were voices crying out for perspective, including mine even before my detailed discussion in *The Last Well Person* in 2004. But entrenched theories such as this can become a "scientific truth" that outlives its critics so that the next generation knows no better. I have no doubt this would have happened if it weren't for the rosiglitazone (Avandia®) canard.

The thiazolidinediones are a new class of oral hypoglycemics that work by sensitizing cells to insulin through a unique biochemistry. Three of these agents have survived the gantlet of clinical trials to be introduced into the marketplace. One, troglitazine, was quickly removed because of toxic effects on the liver, which were too infrequent to be detected in the trials but too frequent to be ignored when widely prescribed. Two remain: rosiglitazone (Avandia®) and pioglitazone (Actos®). Both drive glucose metabolism toward normal at the price of a tendency toward fluid retention. Both held the usual promise of important benefits based only on the theory that normalizing blood glucose was critical; no such benefit could be demonstrated. Nonetheless, GlaxoSmithKline (GSK) marketed rosiglitazone to the tune of some $3 billion in sales before the waters turned troubled in 2007.

Part of the marketing was to underwrite several trials, some that looked at combination therapies and others that were merely seed trials. In 2007 several papers appeared that collected the outcome data from these various trials into statistical models termed meta-analyses. This is an exercise that purports to take advantage of the greater numbers of subjects resulting from the merging of the data in multiple trials. When tens of thousands instead of thousands are exposed, relatively infrequent toxicities can be more readily discerned. What emerged was the strong suggestion that the thiazolidinediones were associated with an increase in the incidence of serious cardiovascular complications, including heart failure, heart attacks, and death. The risk from rosiglitazone was for all of this; for pioglitazine, the risk for death was not demonstrable.[56]

Rosiglitazone did not fare too well when the experience of elderly patients in Ontario was analyzed.[57] But the firestorm was ignited when Steven Nissen and Kathy Wolski published their meta-analysis of forty-two trials in the *New England Journal of Medicine* purporting to show a relative increase of heart attacks and death from cardiovascular causes approaching 50 percent.[58] Remember, this is a relative risk; the absolute risk is quite small but not trivial in a frail population and not readily justified in the absence of any evidence that rosiglitazone leads to any important benefit. The editors of the *New England Journal of Medicine* weighed in, along with essays by multiple experts.[59] They picked at the methods employed in the meta-analysis and looked at the various trials for such biases as recruiting sicker or older subjects and more. Uncertainties about the validity of the cardiovascular adverse effects trumped uncertainties as to the inferences regarding the potential for benefit. Rosiglitazone was not pulled from the market in 2007. Rather, the FDA in the United States and the European Medicines Agency felt that a warning was all that was called for.[60]

Because of this brouhaha, the oversight committee for the RECORD trial felt compelled to report interim results in 2007, long before the six-year trial was completed.[61] RECORD is the acronym for the Rosiglitazone Evaluated for Cardiac Outcomes and Regulation of Glycaemia in Diabetes trial. If nothing else, it's testimony to the pharmaceutical industry's mastery of acronyms. This trial recruited subjects whose blood sugar was well controlled on either of two older drugs and randomized them to a combination of the two older drugs or rosiglitazone. The authors argued that "the findings are important in answering some of the safety concerns raised by the recent meta-analysis by Nissen and Wolski." The two experts who wrote the editorial accompanying the publication of the interim analysis of RECORD were far less certain.[62] Neither Steven Nissen[63] nor the Committee on Finance of the U.S. Senate[64] was willing to let it rest. At the very least, it appears that officials in GSK and scientists/clinicians with financial ties to GSK had been behaving in an unseemly fashion. GSK had unauthorized access to the Nissen-Wolski meta-analysis prior to publication and had meddled with the putatively independent oversight committee for RECORD. Nissen was struck by the relative dearth of adverse cardiovascular events in the final report of RECORD, which was published in 2009, and concerned that academic governance by the trial's steering and oversight committees was compromised because the raw data necessary for an independent analysis was not made available. It gets uglier. GSK was accused of trying to suppress an editorial written by Nissen titled "The rise and fall of rosiglitazone," which saw the light of day nonetheless in the *European Heart Journal*.[65] Subsequently, the European regulatory agencies pulled rosiglitazone from the market. The FDA felt it necessary to waffle. The drug was not withdrawn. Rather, warnings and stringent requirements regarding the indications for its use were applied.

The downside of this firestorm is that it is turning the attention of nearly everyone away from the most important observation. Treating the blood sugar of patients who are labeled type 2 diabetics has not been shown to advantage them despite fifty years of seeking such validation. Furthermore, the quest for this Holy Grail is unabated, with little or no joy from using the available drugs in new combinations or with more aggressive dosing;[66] in fact, these trials suggest we can do more harm without doing any good.[67] If there is nothing good happening, how can the medical establishment and the FDA countenance any hint of doing harm? All oral hypoglycemics should be taken off the market until one can be shown to benefit some group of patients, any group of patients. That's obvious—so why hasn't it happened? One answer is that there is such a cloud of smoke and so many mirrors that too few see clearly to join me in this outcry. Another answer is greed.

The oral hypoglycemic scam swims in money and is promulgated by pervasive conflictual relationships. Let's start with the medical experts, often called "thought leaders," and the doctors involved in recruiting their patients into all these trials. As an example, the American Association of Clinical Endocrinologists and the American College of Endocrinology convened a "consensus panel," which published "an algorithm for glycemic control" in type 2 diabetes.[68] In other words, twelve experts brought the science (which we just summarized) and their preconceptions to the table and came up with their recommendations for treating "high" blood sugar. Of course, by now you can guess at the recommendations. Would you also guess that each of the twelve declared financial arrangements with companies involved in purveying the very pharmaceuticals they were recommending: consultancies, research grants, honoraria for speaking, equity arrangements, and so on. The number of such varied between seven and twenty-seven. Other panels representing other professional organizations but comprised of similarly intertwined "thought leaders" are racing to promulgate minor variations of the same "lower the blood sugar" theme in response to the rosiglitazone/RECORD controversy—the American Diabetes Association, for example.[69]

Amy Wang and Christopher McCoy are residents training in internal medicine at the Mayo Clinic. Along with Professors Mohammad Murad and Victor Monton, they decided to explore the links between published statements on the risk/benefit ratio of rosiglitazone and the declared potential financial conflicts of interest of the authors.[70] They had a rich data set: over 200 commentaries had been published. Half of these papers had a conflict-of-interest statement, and ninety authors volunteered such information. Authors who had financial arrangements with manufacturers of hypoglycemic agents were over six times more likely to come up with an assessment favorable to rosiglitazone than authors who lacked conflictual arrangements. Wang and her coauthors did not attempt to assess conflictual relationships in papers that lacked reporting of such or to validate the information when it was reported. I agree with their assumption that underreporting was likely.

I could easily write a book on the moral compass of thought leaders; I am on record for being intolerant of any conflict of interest on the part of treating physicians, whether they are cognizant of such or just should be cognizant of such.[71] Before you come away with the notion that Dr. Steven Nissen, a cardiologist and the director of the Cleveland Clinic Coordinating Center for Clinical Research, rides the whitest of horses, here's his "Financial Disclosure": "Dr. Nissen reports that the Cleveland Clinic Coordinating Center for Clinical Research has received research support to perform clinical trials from Pfizer, AstraZeneca, Sankyo, Takeda, Sanofi-aventis, Lilly, Roche, Daiichi-Sankyo, and Novartis. Dr. Nissen consults for many pharmaceutical companies, but requires them to donate all honoraria or consulting fees directly to charity so that he receives neither income nor a tax deduction."[72]

The Cleveland Clinic is a nonprofit foundation that generates some $4 billion in annual revenues. In the early 1990s, Dr. Eric Topol was recruited from the University of Michigan to develop what became the 15,000-square-foot "Cardiovascular Coordinating Center" devoted largely to contracting with pharmaceutical firms to undertake drug trials. Topol was chief academic officer and sat on the Clinic's "conflict-of-interest" Committee and Board of Governors. Topol was the academic investigator who spearheaded the assault on Merck for purveying Vioxx without revealing its potential for cardiotoxicity. It turns out that Topol was advising a hedge fund that profited from the decline in Merck stock that resulted from the Vioxx debacle. The clinic stripped Topol of his provost title and unseated him — but do not worry about Dr. Topol. His next stop was a professorship at Case Western Reserve Medical School and on to Scripps Clinic, where he continues to coordinate therapeutic trials. Topol was succeeded by Dr. Nissen as director of what is now called the "Cleveland Clinic Coordinating Center for Clinical Trials"; Dr. Nissen continued in that role until 2005, when he moved into another administrative position at the clinic.

I have no reason to doubt Dr. Nissen's "disclosure," but medical directors of "Contract Research Organizations" are generally very well compensated, reflecting the profitability of their center's contractual relationships with industry. For example, Dr. Nissen headed up an $800 million study of a Pfizer drug to alter blood lipids. He also headed up the $100 million post-marketing PRECISION study that provided the shakiest of scientific grounds for the FDA to preserve the license for Pfizer's Celebrex, then the only remaining competitor for Merck's Vioxx.

What goes around comes around; another "thought leader" cardiologist, Valentin Fuster, wrote a critique of Nissen's work on rosiglitazone in *Nature Clinical Practice Cardiovascular Medicine*. Fuster was receiving

GSK funding and served as the chairman of GSK's Research and Education Foundation. I personally don't find this a "boys will be boys" moment. I share some of the hesitancy to declare Nissen a Nadaresque figure that Stephanie Saul expressed in a July 27, 2007, *New York Times* essay. She was commenting on whether donating "consultancy" fees to charity mollifies the conflictual nature of the arrangement: "Beneficiaries of the money, hundreds of thousands of dollars over the years, have included the American College of Cardiology. Another recipient has been the Cleveland Museum of Art, one of the major museums and galleries that has shown the work of his wife, Linda Butler, an award-winning photographer." All this was before Nissen became president of the American College of Cardiology.

Enough about Nissen; let's examine the notion of a Contract Research Organization (CRO). The Cleveland Clinic Coordinating Center for Clinical Research is one of many examples of CROS housed in hospitals and medical schools. The industry, however, was developed first as a freestanding enterprise. I know a lot about CROS since the first, and the largest, is Quintiles Transnational, which was founded by a colleague, academic collaborator, and coauthor when we were both junior faculty at the University of North Carolina. Dennis Gillings was in the Department of Biostatistics in our School of Public Health, which now bears his name. The industry still has North Carolina for its epicenter, with both Duke and UNC now providing competition by housing their CROS. Gillings's idea to outsource drug trials and licensing applications was attractive to the pharmaceutical industry and has flowered into an industry that offers employment to tens of thousands in America and beyond.

Gillings's is a great American rags-to-riches story. But I have been a vocal critic of this industry from the get-go because I consider it inherently conflictual and therefore ethically compromised. When we do science, we start with a null hypothesis and do our best to refute the hypothesis. The null hypothesis is that the drug doesn't work. If we reject this null hypothesis, the deduction that the drug works is as valid as the rigor with which we tested the null hypothesis. And even if we are impressed with the rigor, we remain uncertain about the degree to which our testing was rigorous. A scientist always worries about confounders that weren't or couldn't be measured and biases that were stealth.

Science tries to disprove any hypothesis and offers tentative positive conclusions when it fails to do so. CROS are contracted by industry to do science, but the hope is always that the hypothesis (the drug doesn't work) will be rejected. In fact, no pharmaceutical firm contracts a CRO to study a drug without fervently hoping for a positive result. The pharmaceutical firm is not paying a fortune for some CRO to do everything possible to pull the rug out from under its latest potential source of profit. Since most drug trials are seeking small effects with large populations, the rigorousness of the testing and data analysis is critical. Small lapses in the collection or interpretation of data can make a difference, and small lapses are the rule. For the scientist, the ethic is to prejudice the analysis toward *not* rejecting the null hypothesis that the drug doesn't work. For the CRO, the push-back to this ethic is neither trivial nor subtle. A contracting pharmaceutical firm that is disappointed too frequently by one CRO and not another is reflexively likely to feel an affinity for the productive relationship. These trials are too important to be handled in a cloud of prejudicial science. The RECORD trial is the handiwork of the UK subsidiary of Quintiles Transnational.

GSK is not even close to abandoning its cash cow, rosiglitazone. In 2007 GSK contracted for the Thiazolidinedione Intervention in Vitamin D Evaluation (or TIDE trial). This is a randomized controlled trial that the FDA ordered GSK to conduct in response to the controversy "to test the cardiovascular effects of long-term treatment with rosiglitazone or pioglitazone when used as part of standard of care." There are nearly 140 sites in fourteen countries, including in resource-disadvantaged countries, trying to accumulate 16,000 subjects. It's another of the many JUPITER-like trials that support an enormous industry but offer no likelihood of benefit for those among us who will subsidize all this sophistry in the cost of pills and the price of "health" insurance. The FDA ordered enrollment in TIDE to cease in the summer of 2010 and discontinued the trial soon thereafter.

I introduced this discussion of rosiglitazone with the 2008 Recommendations of the USPSTF to screen for type 2 diabetes in hypertensive patients because the hypertension in patients with type 2 diabetes is "more dangerous and more responsive" to antihypertensive therapy. Yes, it is more dangerous; but the assertion that it is more responsive to therapy was on shaky ground. That's why the National Institutes of Health felt justified in underwriting the ACCORD studies; the acronym stands for Action to Control Cardiovascular Risk in Diabetes. Over 10,000 patients with type 2 diabetes treated in a standard fashion were recruited into a complex protocol testing the benefit of more intensive treatment of blood glucose, blood pressure, and blood lipids. The first study made it into the Nissen analysis for increased cardiotoxicity. The results of the last two of these large multicenter studies were recently published. Five years of attempting to drive the systolic blood pressure below 135–140 offered no important advantage in terms of death, heart attack, or stroke but did lead to a doubling of the incidence of serious adverse events attributed to the antihypertensive treatment.[73] It also didn't matter if they pummeled blood cholesterol.[74]

When will we ever learn? There is a forest and there are trees. Lowering glucose is the wrong tree.[75]

Hypertension

I see people sticking their arms into blood pressure (BP) cuffs wherever I go—my gym, many a drugstore, and of course the "check-in" by the nurses in the clinic. I know of many people who feel remiss if they don't weigh themselves each day and follow that with a blood-pressure measurement. These metrics have commandeered our concept of life nearly to the extent that time has done. Time took millennia to do so; BP took one generation.

When we discussed BMI, I demonstrated that the risk-for-death curve was a flat-based U. There was no increased likelihood for death before your time if your BMI was greater than 18.5 and less than 35 unless you were also poor, miserable, angry, or otherwise uncomfortable in your skin.

When we discussed blood cholesterol, I suggested a similar image, a U-shaped curve for risk—though the risk imparted by "high" cholesterol in the population at large does not approach the risk of morbid obesity, except in the extreme examples of families with genetic disorders of cholesterol metabolism. Nonetheless, we live with the mandate for lowering cholesterol and the daunting realization of "so what." The lesson was that cholesterol was a minor risk factor and treating "high" cholesterol in well people was nectar for the pharmaceutical industry and sophistry for the treated. Treating high cholesterol in older well people is unconscionable.

Hypertension merits similarly close attention. There are two general categories of hypertension. That which most people get is called "essential hypertension," and that which is associated with diseases, particularly with kidney diseases, is called "secondary hypertension" because it is secondary to an underlying disease. This second category is very different and demands a very different mindset on the part of patients and physicians. It is one of the reasons I will advocate the occasional visit to your primary-care physician, someone who should know who you are as you age and who knows that you are not harboring kidney disease if your blood pleasure is up. When my patients with lupus or scleroderma trend toward hypertension, it signals kidney involvement, and I pull out all the stops in treating their hypertension. People and patients with essential hypertension deserve a reasoned discussion of benefits and risks before engaging in an assault on their blood pressure. Such a discussion is hampered by scientific uncertainties.

First, there is a problem with this dichotomy. Some people with essential hypertension go on to, or already have, kidney disease. These people are in a vicious cycle of escalating blood pressure, which causes kidney disease to occur or progress, which causes further escalation in the blood pressure. It is for fear of this vicious cycle that physicians have been instructed for decades to treat a patient with essential hypertension to normalize their blood pressure. As the clinical science has matured, it turns out that nothing about this topic has proved straightforward, particularly as it relates to people in their Golden Years and after. We are learning that discordance between blood pressure and kidney scarring is far more common than a vicious cycle between them.

The kidney's function is to clean the blood of the toxic waste products of metabolism. Nearly all of us are born with about four times the minimum kidney capacity necessary to do this and stay well. The strongest predictor of diminished capacity is age. Capacity is diminished in about 4 percent of people aged twenty to forty and about 50 percent of people over age seventy. Fortunately, this decrease in capacity seldom reaches the critical level that causes one to be ill from kidney failure, although kidney side effects of drugs are more likely to be manifest in these elderly patients. If we were to biopsy the usual elderly patient whose kidney is failing, the microscopic picture is one of scarring of the working components of the tissue, so-called nephrosclerosis. Since nearly all elderly patients with kidney failure from nephrosclerosis also have high blood pressure, it has long been assumed that high blood pressure caused nephrosclerosis and that treating high blood pressure spared the kidney from nephrosclerosis. It turns out that mild-to-moderate nephrosclerosis is not rare in perfectly well people with normal blood pressures.[76] The prevalence rises from 16 percent in our twenties to 60 percent in our sixties and 70 percent in our seventies. Risk factors such as high blood pressure do not account for the prevalence of nephrosclerosis. It may account for its progression, but the relationship between blood pressure and kidney disease is tenuous. It must be that there is something else going on, some factor other than hypertension that we have yet to identify. Treating hypertension to spare the kidney is a flawed, wizened axiom.

Just as nephrosclerosis is an aging phenomenon, so too is "high blood pressure." We are all aware of the age-related decrease in the rigor with which collagen keeps our skin taught. But we are not aware that the firmness of our major blood vessels is going the other way at the same time. The large vessels are more rigid, meaning they are less compliant and therefore less able to expand when the heart pumps the next bolus of blood into the tube. The result is a higher systolic pressure and a lower diastolic pressure. In fact, it would be abnormal if the systolic-diastolic difference (called the pulse pressure) didn't widen in our Golden Years. We are running the risk of medicalizing normal aging when we define "high" blood pressure. Labeling someone hypertensive is justifiable only if it has been demonstrated that blood pressure imparts more information than age alone or that treating putatively "high" BP leads to some meaningful advantage for the person.

The association between hypertension and heart attack, stroke, or important kidney disease is more J-shaped than U-shaped, with the J lying on its side so that the slope is shallow:

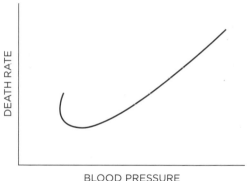

BLOOD PRESSURE

Hence, there is relatively little increase in risk for a given increase in blood pressure until a dangerous threshold is reached. Equally daunting is the fact that treating "high" blood pressure drives one back down the shallow J-shaped risk curve until, unpredictably, one is driven up the portion where adverse outcomes escalate rapidly. Treating essential blood pressure, particularly in the elderly, is a double-edged sword with neither side uniformly honed.

On that background, we are asked to applaud the fact that hypertension was "controlled" in about half of all patients with hypertension in

2008.[77] Is this reason to celebrate? Is this reason to bemoan the fate of the other half? Or do we need to step back and ask what we've accomplished?

Yes, there are august committees such as the Joint National Committee on which sit august professionals charged with looking at the epidemiology of blood pressure and defining "high." All are invited because they are convinced that essential hypertension is not simply a surrogate marker of risk for cardiovascular disease but an important causal factor, if not actually a disease itself. For these believers, it follows that smiting hypertension a mighty blow will advantage the people who are at risk far more than those involved in the purveyance of the smiting. For about a decade, the definition of hypertension in the "Seventh Report" of the Joint National Committee held sway: hypertension is diagnosed by a systolic pressure of 140 mm of mercury (Hg) or a diastolic pressure of 90mm Hg or greater. These limits were deduced by an analysis of the experience in the Framingham, Massachusetts, study in which thousands of people are followed for decades. By this definition, more than 90 percent of people who have a normal BP at age fifty-five will develop hypertension as they age. Once beyond the 140/90 boundaries, some of these aging people are at increasing *risk* as their blood pressure climbs up the gentle slope of the reclining J-shaped curve. However, at any level in this climb, a substantial proportion of the population has no increased risk.[78] Treating in such a circumstance is a setup for doing more harm than good.

I've been hammering home the principle that one never wants to be screened for anything unless the test is accurate, the disease is important, and we can do something of substance for you if you screen positive. Well, we all know that BP readings are quite variable. The usual compromise is to define hypertension as elevated readings on at least two occasions separated by a week or so. Whether one considers it a surrogate marker or a causal factor, hypertension speaks to an increment in risk of cardiovascular disease, and that's important. Furthermore, we have been able to lower BP with drugs for half a century with the presumption that we lower risk by so doing. No wonder the USPSTF recommends screening for high blood pressure.[79]

I've also been hammering home the principle that one should never assume that treating a surrogate measure such as BP actually reduces your risk to a meaningful degree. Treating hypertension is big business, with many classes of drugs flooding the marketplace in waves. All on the market are licensed by the FDA because the agency was convinced that the drug actually lowers BP without undue short-term toxicities. None are licensed because of data showing that a meaningful reduction in untoward cardiovascular outcomes results over time. However, a massive amount of such data has accumulated; one review collected over 147 randomized prospective trials seeking such an effect.[80] Most failed to discern benefit in the long term, although the authors of many of these studies massage their data to conform to their preconceptions or spin their negative results.[81] Some of the most famous and influential demonstrated the potential for harm from treating hypertension; two were stirring the pot long before we entered the twenty-first century.

"MR FIT," the first, is the acronym for the Multiple Risk Factor Intervention Trial.[82] Over 350,000 men age thirty-three to forty-seven were screened in 1973 and followed for over twenty-five years. If they developed hypertension, they were treated with "step therapy" starting with older drugs with little toxicities and adding agents until BP was normalized. One of the oldest and mildest of the drugs is a thiazide-class of diuretic. In MR FIT, exposure to this agent was associated with increased likelihood of an adverse cardiovascular outcome, including death.

The second, "ALLHAT," is the acronym for the Antihypertensive and Lipid-Lowering Treatment to Prevent Heart Attack Trial. This was a comparison of treatment regimens in 42,000 people: an inexpensive generic thiazide-class agent and three expensive agents of distinctive newer classes (an ACE inhibitor, a calcium channel blocker, and an alpha blocker). The last option proved toxic and was removed from the trial. The thiazide-class agent outperformed the remaining two. These data have been sliced and diced repeatedly over the past decade since the main results were published in 2002. There is no way to escape the inference that a gentle thiazide-based intervention is the first-line pharmaceutical approach to managing essential hypertension.[83]

So, MR FIT suggests staying away from the thiazide-class as initial therapy for hypertension, and ALLHAT says it's apple pie. The dissonance can be explained by an important variable, a confounder that went unmeasured in the initial analysis of the MR FIT data because it was not well known to be important. It just happens that more of the volunteers treated with a thiazide were drawn from a lower socioeconomic stratum. Correcting for this confounder exonerates thiazides, even in MR FIT.[84] Multiple other studies reach a similar conclusion. If one decides to treat essential hypertension, a low-dose thiazide is the most defensible first-line approach.[85]

In the twenty-first century, the thrust of many randomized trials has shifted to address several hotly debated issues, with a great deal of pharmaceutical largesse at play in the debate. To start, should essential hypertension be treated with any pharmaceuticals? This is the argument that has come to the fore, usually under the banners of "lifestyle change," dietary restrictions, and salt restriction. Much of this is playing out in a younger population or subpopulation that has the "metabolic syndrome": increased BMI, abnormal blood lipids, and elevated BP (and generally lower socioeconomic status). When it comes to hypertension, until recently the thrust was pharmacological. But now, dietary modification is touted for this component of the metabolic syndrome—mainly salt restriction.[86] The notion has caught on in public-health circles, been sanctioned by the Institute of Medicine, and caught the eye of Congress. It is argued forcibly that we should get the salt out of our food chain, get dietary intake down to some 2g/day, and we would do wonders for the health of the public. As you know from the preface, wise clinicians have thought little of a 2g/day sodium diet in the past. And one very wise and very experienced renowned expert in hypertension, Michael Alderman, is calling for caution today.[87] Some of Alderman's arguments are familiar at this point since they reiterate our discussions above regarding surrogate outcomes and missing the forest for the trees. Alderman points out that one of the randomized controlled trials of dietary salt restriction in patients with heart failure demonstrated harmfulness from overzealous restriction. More important, there have been over a dozen observational cohort studies in which groups were followed for some time and clinical outcomes correlated with their salt consumption. The results have been conflicting. Alderman attempted to make mathematical sense of this hodgepodge. He argues that the risk of dietary sodium follows a J-shaped curve similar to that of hypertension itself. "Normal" sodium intake hovers closer to 4g/day and not the 2g/day that the health policy folks are now trying to promote. Alderman's "normal" can be achieved by caution with the salt shaker rather than reformulating all food preparation.

If treated pharmacologically, should BP be normalized with additional agents if the thiazide alone does not normalize it? The results of randomized trials addressing this question have been very inconsistent. Most trials that add drug after drug to normalize BP are not encouraging.[88] And there's more than a little smoke about the harm in doing so.[89]

Finally, since BP is a risk factor along the continuum of the upward-sloping J-shaped curve, shouldn't patients be treated to get their BP as low as possible, even below the "normal" of 140/90? The Cochrane Collaboration found seven randomized controlled trials that were considered to be of sufficient quality to address this query and concluded that pushing harder on BP control does not advantage the patients.[90] Meanwhile, a group of investigators who do these trials found thirty-one trials to be informative, not just the Cochrane's seven, and reached the opposite conclusion.[91] There is much at stake for the pharmaceutical industry if "tight control" dies on an evidentiary sword. A subsequent attempt to find a benefit took advantage of a subset of 6,400 patients with type 2 diabetes who already had symptomatic coronary artery disease and were enrolled in a trial of antihypertensive regimens. The incidence of cardiovascular outcomes did not depend on the tightness of control of blood pressure.[92] Take that, Damocles.

As I said, there is little that is straightforward about the diagnosis and management of essential hypertension. There is no doubt that hypertension is an important risk factor. At the extremes of the spectrum, BP signals imminent catastrophe and demands attempts at intervention. I would argue that a gentle thiazide and gentle dietary sodium restriction represent the state of the therapeutic art for mild or even moderate essential hypertension, and leave it at that. I stand on fairly solid ground with my argument.[93] Others are constantly trying to undermine my fairly solid ground,[94] and maybe someday they'll succeed. However, today I would need a convincing explanation as to benefits and risks before I would be compliant with a more aggressive pharmaceutical or dietary regimen.

A Little Common Stents

I spend many a day on all fours, playing with trains or puzzles or whatever with one or another or several of our toddling or even older grandchildren. Often, across the room and also on all fours, is their other grandfather. When I was a child, such a scene was unlikely. One or both grandfathers would have died or become decrepit, let alone aloof. In one generation, the structure of the family in the resource-advantaged world has changed thanks to the increased longevity of my birth cohort. We can hope for slightly greater longevity of my children's birth cohort, and, if the resource-advantaged world can figure out a way to be "advanced" instead of just advantaged, a tiny bit greater yet for the grandchildren. That's the implication of the U.S. longevity curves (Figure 1 in chapter 1), which are plots of age-specific, all-cause mortality.

It is difficult not to be awestruck by such an impressive change in longevity. Of all the killers that plagued my father's generation, none has turned gentler for my generation than cardiovascular disease. The age-adjusted mortality rate from coronary artery disease has decreased over 30 percent, from numbers such as 200 deaths per 100,000 people per year to 125. The queue of peoples who are taking credit for this happy turn of events is quite long. In Ontario, about half the improvement is ascribed to improvement in risk factors and medical treatments.[95] In Finland, getting the potatoes off of their couches is applauded.[96] In the UK, it's the decrease in health-adverse behaviors.[97] But then the Scots realized that all these "good" things were surrogate measures of relative wealth. The poor are mired in a bad prognosis to which they are prone to add health-adverse behaviors.[98] Alistair Leyland offers what I consider an understatement: "deliberate interventions to reduce inequalities in health through modification of major risk factors have had limited success to date."[99] As we've reviewed, even if folks are compliant with all the health-promotion advice, the yield is small to nil. The secret to longevity is the structure of society, not whether anyone eats bran. If you are still not convinced, return to chapter 1.

More particularly, the dramatic reduction in age-adjusted mortality from cardiovascular disease cannot be ascribed to the trumpeted and headlined technical wizardry of modern interventional cardiology and cardiovascular surgery. It is true that the reduction in the risk-standardized mortality rate from acute myocardial infarction in patients covered by Medicare has paralleled the reduction in all-cause mortality.[100] The five-year mortality for a well man after his first heart attack has dropped from 50 percent to 5 percent in one generation. The line of people who are taking credit for this happy turn of events is even longer, and many have diamond pinky rings. Celebrities extol their life-saving surgeons and interventional cardiologists, who in turn join them strutting on the world stage. If you have survived one of these modern medical miracles unscathed, there is no way to process the experience other than by proclaiming you were blessed to live in such a medically advantaged community. If symptoms return, it seems so reasonable to return to this technological fountain. If you survived scathed, there is no way to process the experience but to agree that even modern medical miracles were no match for the magnitude of your affliction. And if you didn't survive, your survivors have only your disease to blame.

This is the social construction that every American has been taught and nearly every American has accepted. I have been decrying this sophism in lectures and in print throughout all the decades it took for it to become common wisdom. I started out relying on first principles, but as the technology evolved, so did the clinical science testing its efficacy. There is no doubt in my mind that interventional cardiology and cardiovascular surgery for coronary artery disease has written the bleakest chapter in the entire history of Western medicine.

I detail much of this in *Worried Sick*, starting with the dismal history of Coronary Artery Bypass Graft (CABG) surgery and moving on to the ever-more-dismal history of angioplasty and stenting. CABG is major surgery fraught with complications in the short and long term. It is a procedure where a conduit is fashioned around some major blockage in a vessel that nurtures the heart muscle (and sometimes several vessels). In angioplasty, a catheter with a balloon tip is inserted via the artery into the blockage and the balloon is inflated, tearing the blockage asunder. Blood vessels are not happy with either procedure and have a tendency to clot and permanently reocclude. To decrease that likelihood following angioplasty, metal conduits (stents) are left behind in the lumen of the disrupted vessel. But the body does not look kindly on foreign materials lodged in its blood vessels. Stents like to clot, too. To decrease the likelihood of reocclusion, these stents are often coated with various chemicals and drugs. I freely admit that the technical and technological prowess that has been recruited to this effort is awesome. Likewise, the industry that supports the performance of well over a million such procedures a year in the United States is not simply sizable, it's a behemoth.

So why am I so exercised? Because many systematic studies have been undertaken that were designed to demonstrate that doing any sort of violence to coronary arteries advantages the patient more than pills and other medical therapies. None of these studies, not a one, can demonstrate benefit of stenting to the patient. No patient is rewarded in terms of longevity, incidence of heart attacks, or likelihood of chest pain for having submitted to these expensive technical and technological feats, and many suffer harm in the course of the procedure.

For example, there are a growing number of trials comparing medical therapy with angioplasty/stenting in carefully chosen groups of patients for whom angioplasty was considered a reasonable option. Here are my picks as the best of the lot. None can find an advantage to invasive therapy.

- In the RITA-2 trial, 1,000 carefully selected patients with angina in 1997 were randomized to angioplasty or medical therapy. The

consequences were last reported in 2003. Those initially randomized to noninvasive treatment did as well as those who underwent
angioplasty.[101]

- Angioplasty was invented by a Swiss cardiologist. Subsequently,
Swiss investigators randomized patients over age seventy-five with
angina to optimized medical therapy or early invasive therapy with
angioplasty ± stent or CABG and followed them for four years. There
was no advantage to the early invasive strategy in terms of death or
myocardial infarction.[102]

- The COURAGE trial is particularly damning; no one with stable
angina should be told that angioplasty, with or without stenting,
prevents a heart attack or stroke or prolongs life.[103]

- In a multicenter trial funded by the National Institutes of Health,
2,000 patients were recruited within a month of their heart attack
because they had persistent blockage of the relevant coronary artery
and heart damage. All received optimal medical care; half were
randomized to also undergo angioplasty and stent placement. Over
the next four years, there was no difference between the two groups
in terms of recurrent heart attack, death, or heart failure. If anything,
those with the stents fared less well.[104]

- Even if the comparison is with high-risk patients with type 2 diabetes, there is no advantage to prompt revascularization over medical
therapy for coronary artery disease.[105]

If a physician were ever to say to me that coronary artery disease may be
causing my symptoms, I would listen attentively. If the physician went
on to advise defining my coronary artery "anatomy" by stress testing or
coronary angiography, I would demur. Knowing me and my knowledge of
this decision tree, I would probably not be polite in so doing; I'm likely to
get in that physician's face with, "You've got to be kidding!" Of course, I'd
expect the reader to be more polite. However, I'd hope any reader would
be sufficiently informed to query, "To what end?"

There is no response based on scientific data other than this: despite
trying repeatedly, we can't show the benefit of doing more to you than
prescribing some pills. That is an unequivocal assertion for saving your
life or sparing you a heart attack, and it is rapidly becoming an unequivocal statement for sparing you symptoms.[106] Furthermore, the best data
for "some pills" is with low-dose aspirin, particularly during and after a
heart attack. If you've never had symptoms that are ascribed to coronary

artery disease, it's very difficult to demonstrate any benefit from low-dose aspirin therapy.[107] Prescribing any other agent to interfere with blood clotting, such as clopidogril (Plavix), is buying into the most marginal of benefit/risk ratios. And other commonly prescribed drugs, such as beta blockers, ACE inhibitors, and statins, are testimony to the American philosophy of "don't just stand there, do something" rather than evidence-based, informed medical decision making. The benefit/risk ratio of CABG and angioplasty is zero since we can't demonstrate any benefit. There is a tiny subset with a particular blockage that might be benefited by CABG, but this hardly justifies pushing the vast majority through the risks of cardiac catheterization to identify this tiny subset.

So why is it that over a million such invasive procedures are performed in the United States each year and indemnified by all private insurers, all Medicaid programs, and Medicare? If angioplasty was a pharmaceutical, do you think the FDA could find a way to license it when the critical data prerequisite to licensing a drug was a series of negative randomized controlled trials? But procedures are not subjected to licensing, and devices such as stents are held to a much lower standard; they must be safe in the short term, but there need not be a demonstration of efficacy. Hence, the FDA is not standing between Americans and the invasive cardiology and cardiovascular surgery community. Since the coronary-artery plaque-removal enterprise is the recipient of a sizable portion of the "health-care dollar," it has the fiscal wherewithal to make certain that it is favored in the media, in Congress, and generally in the mind of the public. A few of the leading medical journalists, such as John Carey,[108] have had the editorial support to display the relevant science as early as 2005, but such efforts are overwhelmed by the miasma of marketing.

How about the doctors who do this violence to our coronary arteries? The "thought leaders" are well aware of this science. But most can overcome my kind of compunctions with three rationales.

One I call the "folly of peer review." These interventional cardiologists and cardiovascular surgeons have invested a great deal of time in gaining the skills necessary to assault coronary arteries. They are treated with adulation and largesse by their hospitals and by other aspects of the "health-care" industry that depends on them. They are prominent in their communities, where their incomes, if nothing else, command respect. It is human nature for such people to come together bursting with pride that "my stent is bigger than your stent." It is not human nature to applaud the "peer" who questions whether the stenting should have been done in the first place. The folly of peer review is not exclusive to my guild; it operates widely, including on Wall Street, when wizards were bundling bigger junk mortgages.

Another rationale is science based. All randomized controlled trials specify the population that is recruited. Criteria include such elements as age, coincidental diseases, prior cardiac history, current symptoms, and the like. It is easy for an interventionalist to tell a patient that he or she is different from the subjects in the studies and that, "In my experience, this works for patients like you." For all I know, the interventionalist is correct—but believing so is a matter of faith in the face of the precedent that medical therapy works better in all other circumstances. For me, creating a theory that is self-serving is the essence of quackery. Any such theory should be subjected to testing before it can or should be offered based "on my experience."

The third rationale is an example of massaging scientific data and spinning negative results. If you go to an American emergency room with chest pain, everything will be done to get you to the cardiac catheterization laboratory as quickly as possible and on to angioplasty (± stent) or CABG if the eyes of the beholding interventionalist are convinced it's feasible. They are in such a hurry because it's so difficult to demonstrate that you are better off for the procedure(s) if there is any delay. Since it is believed that the procedures are inherently sensible, it follows that they should be done as quickly as possible. Across the country, and increasingly elsewhere in the world, "algorithms" (road maps) are the standard of care for conditions such as chest pain, which stipulate the steps a physician is to take to make a presumptive cardiac diagnosis and then follow the putatively best course of treatment. The result is that there is little if any time to make an informed medical decision; the decision process is co-opted by the putatively emergent nature of the intervention. Rather than give up on this approach to the acute heart attack, admitting that the likelihood of a good outcome is certainly not dramatically improved (if at all) by racing to open the vessel, the rallying cry is, "Don't delay even an hour or two or it won't work." In fact, in some studies you are better off if your local hospital lacks a cardiac catheterization laboratory, thus sparing you from this vortex. Why are we sharing the cost of any of this? (Yes, we share the cost since indirectly our income underwrites the tens of billions of dollars of indemnity costs.) We are mortgaging our country to support an industry that scorns scientific rigor. That's irrational.

Speaking of scientific testing, I find it striking that interventional cardiology and cardiovascular surgery offers no advantage over medical therapy in terms of symptoms for so many clinical subsets. "Interventions" that are dramatic tend to have an enormous placebo effect because the providers exude enthusiasm, the recipients drip preconceptions of benefit, and the result is colored by the need for justification by both parties. I would have thought that the only way to test the efficacy of interventional procedures such as CABG and angioplasty for chest pain was by randomizing volunteers to the procedure or to a sham procedure. An example of a sham-controlled trial would be where the balloon is inserted into the blockage but only blown up in half the patients. A sham surgery trial was done many years ago for an early version of CABG for severe angina, with a negative result; all patients were anesthetized and all had a skin incision, but only half had the actual bypass performed. The fact that invasive interventions and noninvasive treatments are indistinguishable in so many randomized controlled trials in the setting of symptomatic coronary artery disease makes me wonder if the invasive options are actually harmful, causing patients to cope with more symptoms than otherwise. Of course, these considerations apply to the improvement in symptoms; for "hard" outcomes such as death or heart attacks, placebo effects are not at issue. In all of these trials, invasiveness does no better than medical therapy in saving lives or sparing heart attacks for every form of coronary artery disease that has been studied. I will assume that holds for every form of coronary artery disease that has yet to be studied until a well-designed randomized controlled trial convinces me otherwise. I have been pleading for years for the FDA to pummel the world of devices and techniques with similar sentiments.

For the time being, stenting has taken on a life of its own. The coronary arteries are not the only arteries that can get clogged with atherosclerotic plaques. Those that do so frequently (and that are thought to cause illness) are the carotid arteries to the brain (stroke), the artery to the kidney (a special kind of high blood pressure), the arteries to the legs (foot ulcers and gangrene), and some others. Of course, as is the case for the coronary arteries, when the large arteries are in trouble, so are the smaller arteries downstream. This may explain why interventional cardiology and CABGs don't work; what's the good of opening up the main vessel if the blood doesn't reach the tissue anyway? Vascular surgeons don't seem to have this nightmarish thought; there are surgical procedures to replace blocked carotids, renal arteries, femoral arteries, and more. All of them are dangerous, particularly in the elderly (who are the usual candidates), and none of them are without controversy as to effectiveness. But all of these vessels can be unblocked by angioplasty, reducing, though not eliminating, the procedural risks. Enamored with this technological improvement, interventionalists are leaping to the challenge long before there is data as to whether the patient is benefited in some substantial way. They are not benefited by angioplasty of the carotid arteries,[109] in part because busting the vessel sprays debris downstream, causing strokes despite widgets placed in the vessel to catch the debris. Stenting a blocked artery to the kidney does no good either.[110]

Perhaps the most instructive of the stenting escapades is for a large abdominal aortic aneurism (AAA). The aorta is the large main vessel that leaves the heart and courses down the back into the belly, giving off branches along the way. It, too, always gets atherosclerotic plaques as we age, but unlike other places where occlusion is the hazard, the wall of the aorta tends to weaken and expand into a balloonlike aneurism. In some, particularly in elderly men who smoked, the aneurism grows so large that it bursts. If you get to the hospital before you die, a ruptured AAA is a surgical emergency, but the surgery is very difficult, with lots of complications waiting to happen and unhappy outcomes the rule. So we have long taught that doctors should feel deeply into the abdomen for a pulsating aneurysm and define its size so that if it's getting ripe, it can be repaired electively. Physicians exercise judgment in this regard because even the elective surgical procedure is a big deal and very risky in a frail population. Then some clever people figured out a way to anchor a large stent in the middle of the aneurism, creating a new channel that relieves the fragile wall of the aorta from the pressure of the blood. All of a sudden, it was argued that screening the elderly with ultrasound for an AAA should be undertaken so that any sizable AAA could be stented. The British were not so certain about this argument and undertook a multicenter randomized controlled trial of surgically repairing or stenting AAAs.[111] Between 1999 and 2004, 1,252 subjects volunteered. Indeed, stenting was the less-dangerous procedure. But the long-term outcome in terms of mortality was the same because the stents developed serious complications over time. We're back to clinical judgment regarding intervening when an AAA is detected.[112] A patient of mine, a famous elderly physician, preferred just observing his expanding AAA rather than suffer through and with the repair; he died, but not from the rupture of his AAA.[113]

Foregoing the Apple on Some Days
to See the Good Doctor

Yes, we're back to clinical judgment on a great deal of health-related issues. "Clinical judgment" is not easy to define, let alone measure. It reflects whatever wisdom one has derived from "seeing it before," the collected anecdotes of one's life in the practice of medicine. It reflects whatever wisdom one is capable of distilling from the narratives of patients who are describing their illness. It reflects one's skillfulness in actively listening and in parsing idioms. It reflects one's skillfulness in teasing secrets from the physical body. It reflects an acute awareness of the science that defines the limits of certainty. It reflects one's need for peer review. And most important, clinical judgment grows out of trustworthiness and the establishment of a trusting relationship with the patient.

I've been training, educating, and mentoring physicians in this context for nearly forty-five years. For all those years, I sought and found the same for myself. The only invaluable aspect of the American "health-care system" is the enormous cadre of physicians who would dearly love to practice according to their conscience. But the American "health-care system" constrains them to practice otherwise. "Clinical judgment" takes time in its acquisition and time in its practice. Time spent in this fashion is not encouraged nor rewarded. As I've said often, if any of the rheumatologists I trained practiced the way I trained them, they would starve. Come the revolution, this will all change. But the changing is slow to arrive thanks to the enormous fiscal investment in the status quo.

I know all this, and so do you. But I urge you to find a physician with clinical judgment while you are well and in your Golden Years. It's not that I place any stock in a periodic health evaluation at any age, with good reason.[114] Certainly "screening" is a flimsy rationale, as will become apparent in the next chapter. You only *need* to go to the doctor when you experience some symptom that exceeds your capacity to cope on your own. But you should go to the doctor for the sake of your physician's clinical judgment as it relates to you. Who are you? What's your risk tolerance? What are your health concerns? If there are options, including end-of-life options, what is your preference? Do you trust this physician? Then when you *need* to go to the doctor, you will have recourse to a physician with clinical judgment and be much better off for the effort in establishing the relationship.

3

STAYIN' ALIVE

Let's assume your sixty-fifth birthday is behind you and your eighty-fifth looms somewhere off in the distance. Let's further assume you are well. As we discussed in chapter 1, eighty-five is a realistic goal in terms of longevity. Longer is wishful thinking, and to stay well much longer than eighty-five is a long shot. It is reasonable to ask whether there is anything you can do or that can be done for/to you that will offer assurance at age sixty-five that you will see you eighty-fifth birthday. In the last chapter, we examined the science that speaks to living well while on the journey to eighty-five. But here, the task is to examine the science that might secure the journey itself.

We are about to commence a discussion of "screening" to detect preclinical, subclinical, asymptomatic diseases that can be removed before they can do you harm. Screening is different from diagnostics. Nothing we will discuss precludes a diagnostic exercise. If you have a question about your health, if you've noticed something that is disquieting, if you have any symptom that you can't dismiss as "It's OK" any longer, than take thee to a doctor and ask for reassurance. Whatever happens next is *not* screening, it's diagnostics. Even if some of the testing utilizes modalities that are commonly used in screening, the same modalities are now invoked for diagnostics. If you have a bloody stool and you and your doctor decide that colonoscopy is the best way to find out why, colonoscopy in that instance is a diagnostic test.

The distinction between screening tests and diagnostic testing is not trivial. The diagnostic test is far more likely to yield useful information because it is pursuing a symptom that increases the likelihood that the feared culprit is indeed the underlying disease. Screening tests are done for no other reason than eminent personages have declared it useful for finding culprits before they are symptomatic. So this chapter is a discussion of whether screening is more beneficial than diagnostics for a number of conditions threatening our longevity after age sixty-five.

Since screening tests are seeking diseases that have yet to cause problems, they are up against much greater odds of actually finding the disease (that is, a true positive). This is a property of the test termed its "sensitivity." Furthermore, the degree to which the early, asymptomatic disease is similar to normal variations is the degree to which the screening test is more likely to find an unimportant coincidental disease or an unimportant normal variant. The chance of finding such a false positive is a property of the test termed "specificity." In order to be useful for screening, a screening test must have substantial sensitivity and specificity. The degree to which the screening misses the disease you care about and finds a disease you could care less about is the degree to which the screening is useless — or worse than useless if it requires further testing (like biopsies) to validate the result.

Screening is an exacting exercise in two other ways: you never want to be screened for a disease that is trivial, and you never want to be screened for a disease about which nothing can be done. The former is a waste of time. The latter leads to "labeling," usually negative labeling; you are feeling well only to learn that there is something lurking. Few of us can shrug that off. My favorite example of negative labeling occurs in pediatrics. Many infants and young children have heart murmurs, which are termed "innocent murmurs of childhood" because they have no clinical significance (the heart functions normally) and they go away as the child grows up. If the pediatrician tells the mother that her child has the "innocent murmur of childhood" and explains its insignificance, one would think the mother would shrug it off. Wrong. That child is likely to be kept home in inclement weather or urged to avoid physically demanding activities. It's negative labeling by proxy.

The Lottery Mindset

Before submitting to a screening test, each of us should make an informed decision as to whether the screening is worthwhile from our own perspective. To do so, we should have a handle on the accuracy of the test — its sensitivity and specificity. We should decide before submitting to the testing whether a positive test is important to us. And if a positive test would be important to us, are we convinced that the available treatment is worth the undertaking? This exercise in informed decision making starts with a quantitative statement of likelihood of yield for each question. With the odds defined, the exercise moves on to a highly subjective appreciation of personal values. How worrisome is the disease to me? How much risk of false positives or useless treatments am I willing to tolerate given the degree to which I find this asymptomatic disease worrisome?

There is a serious cultural impediment to undertaking this rational exercise. I call it the lottery mindset. I don't buy lottery tickets. True, someone will win, and likely walk away with a mind-boggling windfall. That someone may be one in a million, but someone will win. It is so unlikely to be that someone, maybe there's a magical force at play, maybe a gambler's gryphon or a good fairy. Many reasonable Americans must believe in the gambler's gryphon. Some have premonitions, a sense that the gryphon will fend for them in the deepest reaches of improbability, where the powerball hides. None of this is irrational behavior. All understand the probabilities, and most get a rise out of the possibilities. Many states have deemed the purchase of lottery tickets legitimate if not moral, usually because some portion of the proceeds goes to the common good . . . and someone wins.

My choice not to play the lottery is simply my choice; it is not a reproach to those who play. However, in America the psychology of the lottery has been so well inculcated that it commonly makes sense to apply it to another challenging win-lose exercise: betting on our health. It drives the "I know the chance is slim, Doc, but let's go for it" response when we or our loved ones are sick. It also drives many other choices related to our health, including our willingness to undergo screening. In the case of the lottery, we know what we're doing. In the case of winning good health, we are all too often bamboozled.

Let's take a hypothetical example.

A. If I offered you a five-year screening program that had been *systematically studied* and shown to spare one person out of 2,000 screened from death from a particular cancer, would you submit?

B. If I told you it was a safe, painless screening test with no downside, would you submit?

C. If I told you it was a safe, painless screening test but also detected five people who would be treated unnecessarily because the cancer would not have been the cause of their death, would you submit?

Before you sign the permission slip, let's make sure you understand what I've told you. The first assertion has the descriptor "systematically studied." That means the efficacy of the screening test was studied by comparing people who were screened with people who were left to their own devices. That means the referent group had access to usual care, including usual diagnostics. In both groups, tumors were detected that were cured and tumors were missed that were lethal. When the data were analyzed, one extra person among the 2,000 screened was spared death from this tumor. Now, are you willing to go for your scheduled screening? Do you think science can detect this subtle a difference? Aren't you almost as likely to be lucky and be cured without a scheduled screening? That's like winning the lottery without buying the ticket. How about if we toss in D and asked you to pay out-of-pocket instead of sharing the cost of the screening with all of us by virtue of our health-insurance premiums? Do you still think we can find one case in 2,000 people over the course of five years? Ten years?

I have serious doubts that we can measure such a small difference. Even if we were talking about inbred mice, I would have serious doubts because of "randomization errors." Whenever we compare one group with another for some health effect, we have to hope that the groups are comparable except for what we do or don't do to one of the groups — screening versus diagnostics in this hypothetical case. If not, we can be fooled by biases we didn't measure, such as more people susceptible to cancer in one group or another. To overcome such bias, we can randomly assign people to the groups and expect that the unmeasured biases will equalize, and largely they do. But nothing is perfect, and small inequalities can creep in. These are called "randomization errors." Some we can measure, such as if more women randomized to the screening group are elderly compared to the diagnostic group. Randomization errors that are measurable can be compensated for in the statistical analysis. Unmeasured and immeasurable randomization errors are always lurking and always threatening to prejudice the outcome. The only way I feel comfortable that the measured health effect reflects the intervention (screening) and not randomization error is when the likelihood of the health effect (finding the evil tumor early enough to cure it) is substantial. For me, the assertion that screening 2,000 people for five years saved one more life than diagnostics is simply not convincing. How about you? If it is convincing, is it convincing enough to tolerate the downside in C?

Screening to Thwart Death by Breast Cancer

This hypothetical scenario is not so hypothetical; rather, it is a fair approximation of the science of the efficacy of screening all women over age forty-five with annual mammography.[1] Someday, we might be able to identify individuals who are at particularly high risk for whom screening is more efficient. Today, the only known subset is women with strong family histories of gynecologic cancer who carry a particular gene, one of the BRCA genotypes. These women are at high risk. They have such a high probability of developing breast cancer that they are urged to forego screening for prophylactic mastectomies.

Until we can identify other markers of high prior probability, screening mammography will remain a very disappointing test at best. The younger the woman, the more it approaches useless because the likelihood of a true positive is vanishingly rare. That's why the U.S. Preventive Services Task Force (USPSTF) could recommend against routine screening mammography in women under age fifty.[2] The task force also concluded that while the degree of efficacy discussed above justified screening mammography in older women, little if anything would be lost if the screening was every other year instead of annual.[3] I would add that the reason there is little to be lost is that the amount to be gained from mammographic screening at any age with any frequency is trivial, even with digital instead of film mammography.[4] The task force appreciates that there is insufficient data to base a recommendation for or against screening in women over seventy but felt that screening up to age seventy-five was the better part of valor based on theoretical models suggesting that as many as two breast cancer deaths might be averted if 1,000 women were screened into their seventies.[5]

It is time for a reality check. Let's assume that we were to follow 1,000 relatively advantaged North American females from birth to death in the twentieth century and allow them access to screening or diagnostic mammography as they see fit. By the time this cohort turned seventy, 150 would have died, five from breast cancer. Between age seventy and eighty-five, two more women would die from breast cancer, while 170 would die from cardiovascular disease and another 220 from other causes. I've taken very little liberty with the Canadian data in offering up this reality check.[6]

The lesson is one of the themes of my earlier book *Worried Sick*,[7] and it is revisited in chapter 1: increasing the number of octogenarians is a measure of the health of the public, while comforting octogenarians as they die testifies to the public wisdom. If we removed both breasts from every eighty-year-old woman, we would not change the date on any of their death certificates, only the "cause" of death of a very few. If we removed both breasts from all women who are seventy, likewise. No amount of torturing of the data by the USPSTF[8] or others[9] will produce a benefit of screening mammography over age seventy that is clinically meaningful.

My advice to women over seventy, or younger than fifty, is to forego screening but to feel free to consult their physician whenever they have concerns about the health of their breasts (or any other health concerns, for that matter). I'm not sure what should trigger concern aside from something like an inversion of or discharge from the nipple, a change in the skin texture, and other obvious changes. Routine breast self-examination is stymied by all the irregularities one can palpate in the normal breast and leads to no improvement in breast-cancer mortality.[10] The public-health advice regarding the trigger for concern is the euphemism "breast awareness."[11] Let me emphasize that I am not trivializing breast cancer or dismissing the tragedy when a woman of any age dies from breast cancer (or anything else) before her time. Rather, I am explaining why screening mammography does not offer anything of substance over diagnostics in confronting this specter. Counterarguments for screening before fifty or after seventy are based on emotion, not science.

The scientific debate relates to the incremental benefit of screening mammography over diagnostics between fifty and seventy. The scientific debate relates to whether sparing one woman in 2,000 death before her time from breast cancer by screening for decades can be justified given the downsides of unpleasant examinations and of unnecessary procedures, labeling, and treatments. The scientific debate relates to whether sparing one woman in 2,000 death before her time from breast cancer by screening is a health benefit that can even be measured reliably. I argue that screening mammography by any imaging modality currently available offers nothing over diagnostics and should be relegated to the historical archives. I have argued as much in multiple lengthy interviews on National Public Radio, in many a commentary and op-ed, and in detail in previous books[12] long before the science had fully matured. I have lectured to and otherwise informed many a health journalist as to the essence of the debate and the object lesson it represents. All this can be done dispassionately.

However, the scientific debate has been drowned out by a highly emotional debate that renders the object lesson almost inaccessible. There are women, many women, who are convinced that the treatment of their breast cancer was successful because the cancer was detected early enough by screening mammography. For many, the "cancer" was one of the less-malignant varieties that would have showed up in diagnostics or would never have been a problem. For some, the sequence of events following mammography was lifesaving, but nearly all, if not all, of these fortunate few would have had a similar happy outcome left to the usual diagnostic devices available to all of us in deciding to be patients. There are many women who have suffered metastatic disease and who feel guilt for having avoided screening mammograms. There are many women who are faced with breast cancer that was "missed" on mammography, enough of whom bring lawsuits against mammographers to make this the leading malpractice suit in America. For all these women who live with the personal assault of the diagnosis of breast cancer, the intellectual and statistical abstractions regarding the utility of screening seem insulting. For them, for their caring community, and for the public at large, mammography is a lifesaving procedure.

That's why the recommendation of the USPSTF to restrict screening to women over fifty was met with a furiously angry response. "Survivors" of breast cancer that was diagnosed before fifty and people who lost young loved ones to breast cancer cried foul, and more. They were joined by older "survivors" and others who had already been similarly provoked by a front-page story in the New York Times a month before the task force's pronouncement. Gina Kolata's story (October 21, 2009) was titled "Cancer Society, in Shift, Has Concerns on Screenings." Kolata interviewed Dr. Otis Brawley, chief medical officer of the American Cancer Society, regarding the implications of an analysis of the scientific data on the efficacy of mammography that had just been published in the Journal of the American Medical Association,[13] an analysis that is similar to that which I have just put forth. Brawley is quoted as saying, "I'm admitting that American medicine has over promised when it comes to screening. The advantages to screening have been exaggerated." What a bombshell! All American women are raised to believe that screening in general, and mammography in particular, was essential to good health. Now the august American Cancer Society was reneging. The cognitive dissonance was palpable. Members of the task force tried to explain the science. Others, including yours truly,[14] took to the airways trying to explain the science. Dr. Brawley and the American Cancer Society backpedaled. Senator Barbara Mikulski introduced legislation mandating access to mammography.

Mammography instantly became the poster child for the "R-word"—rationing—which is one of the third rails of "health care finance" reform.[15] If one believes that the putative small benefit of screening mammography in women under fifty is real and not a statistical artifact, then one can calculate the cost of every "quality-adjusted life-year" (QALY) gained. The cost of a year gained is nearly $700,000. Or, calculated differently, a decade's worth of mammograms starting in her forties would increase a woman's lifespan by five days—which she could neutralize by riding a bicycle with a helmet for fifty hours.[16] As for women over fifty, screening improves the chance of not dying from breast cancer in the next ten years only from about 991/1,000 to 994/1,000.[17] No such argument is a match for the lottery mindset about mammography: "I don't care how much it costs (if someone else pays) or how unlikely the benefit, if it can save even one life, I want to go for it."

Not even the downsides of mammographic screening are dissuasive. Women who have lived through the experience engendered by a false-positive mammogram suffer long-term adverse consequences; they are less likely to return to physicians with concerns about their breast health and more likely to live with a heightened level of anxiety.[18] There is even concern that the radiation exposure from repeated mammograms may predispose to breast cancer.[19] In addition to all the repeated studies, negative biopsies, and biopsies that demonstrate relatively benign lesions, there are the cancers that are treated unnecessarily. This is what is meant by "overdiagnosis." Some grow so slowly that they would not have been lethal ahead of some other grim reaper. Some breast cancers, even invasive breast cancers, seem to go away without treatment.[20]

There is no question that overdiagnosis occurs and no question that it leads to unnecessary treatment, meaning treatment that does not benefit the woman. The question relates to how often it occurs. Based on an analysis of the literature from Australia, Canada, the United Kingdom, and Scandinavia, one in three breast cancers detected by screening is overdiagnosed.[21] However, while the likelihood of overdiagnosis relates to the screening uptake, age, and other demographic features of the population, the most important factor is the criteria used to declare the mammographic image "normal." Welch[22] suggests that for every woman spared death from breast cancer by screening, two to ten women will be

TABLE 3

Risks and Benefits of Mammography Screening

Benefit: Chance of Dying from Breast Cancer

No screening	5.3/1,000
Screening	4.6/1,000

Harms of Screening:

False positive requiring biopsy	50–200/1,000
Overdiagnosis	1–7/1,000

overdiagnosed and treated needlessly; ten to fifteen will be diagnosed with breast cancer, but this earlier diagnosis will not affect their prognosis because the tumor is very slow growing or already metastatic; and 100 to 500 will have at least one false alarm (proven false by biopsy in half of them).

There is no doubt that "defensive medicine" will bias toward overdiagnosis in the United States given the likelihood of a malpractice suit for a "missed" cancer. Estimates by Esserman, Shieh, and Thompson[23] are even more daunting: 800 women will have to be screened for six years to spare one death from breast cancer, but ninety will have undergone biopsies and twenty-four labeled with cancer if not treated unnecessarily. Steven Woloshin and his colleagues are clinical investigators with a particular interest in how to best explain risk and benefit so as to allow a patient to make an informed medical decision. Table 3 is the fashion in which they express the risks and benefits of undergoing screening mammography every one to two years for ten years, compared to no screening for women age fifty to fifty-nine.[24]

That's an impressive personal price to be paid by hundreds of women so that one more woman in almost 1,500 might be spared death from breast cancer. It is particularly upsetting since for every woman so benefited, ten would undergo surgery, chemotherapy, and/or radiation to no avail. In fact, some forms of chemotherapy and radiation therapy have subtle toxicities that may place these ten "diagnostic" women at risk for death before their time. The possibility that one in 1,500 over a decade will be spared does not approach my limit as to the magnitude of risk that can be reliably detected. All this is much ado about exceedingly little putative benefit and more about potential harm. If the benefit was substantial, this level of risk would be tolerable. Still, women are incensed by the suggestion that screening mammography should no longer be an entitlement.

Screening Mammography as Creed

Entrenched belief systems about "health" and the maintenance of health are part of the human condition. Conceptions of illness and modes of treatment vary over time across cultures and within cultures.[25] Culture is more than the sum of the innate and reflective beliefs and behaviors of the individuals in a group. Rather, there are influences in the summing that alter the reflective beliefs and facilitate the innate. This is a process termed "cultural determinism." At the extreme, it suggests that most notions of truth are "socially constructed."[26] When it comes to notions of health, culture has seldom been monolithic. Medical anthropologists use the term "medical pluralism" to denote that in any culture, at any time, multiple conceptions and multiple treatments for any given illness coexist or even compete for supremacy. Low back pain is a dramatic example of this phenomenon.[27] So is cancer. Cancer superseded untreatable infectious diseases as the most horrifying of disease specters in the middle of the twentieth century. It seems intuitive to ascribe this dialectic to the fact that antibiotics triumphed. However, it is not that simple. True, antibiotics triumphed, but this triumph and coincident evolution of the structure of Western societies allowed diseases of later life to come to the fore. Cancer superseded tuberculosis as the leading evil[28] as more people lived long enough to die from cancer. Heart disease and stroke are feared almost as much, as we discussed in the last chapter.

It follows that if we identify and cure cancer early, before it has spread, we would vanquish the specter. This seemingly logical agenda assumes we can cure the cancer and ignores the fact that we might die anyway of something else at about the same time. These provisos were seldom voiced in the twentieth century, and they are seldom voiced today. Rather, "warning signs" were promulgated and screening became de rigueur, long before the demanding nature of effective screening was understood. The enthusiasm for cancer screening in the United States is unabated.[29]

Clearly, when it comes to breast self-examination and screening mammography (and much more, as we will discuss shortly), we need to be disabused. To do so requires an examination of the language, the semantics that promulgated the sophistry in the first place. First, there is the issue of "medicalese," the use of technical terminology to denote irrelevant, minor, or even normal individual differences.[30] That's how an osteophyte became a bone "spur," and the bone "spur" became a cause of back, neck, shoulder, or knee pain. That's how a "lump" became a "lesion," or a "mass," or "ductal carcinoma in situ" (or its ominous acronym, DCIS), so that breast "cancer" became epidemic. The fact that some women are genetically predisposed to cancer has caused many more women to wrongly view their kinship as stained.[31]

Today, the thoughtless use of "medicalese" is inexcusable. But it is not as reprehensible as torturing scientific data and massaging statistical analyses. Look at Table 3 again. The risk of death from breast cancer is reduced by screening for ten years from 5.3 to 4.6 women out of every 1,000 screened. Less than one woman spared in 1,000 screened for a decade is not a very impressive reduction in *absolute* risk, is it? But 5.3 to 4.6 can also be described as a reduction of 13 percent—a *relative* risk reduction of 13 percent. That is a more compelling statistic, isn't it? If the numbers were 0.75/1,000 deaths screened and 1.5/1,000 not screened, that would be almost the same *absolute* risk reduction, but the *relative* risk reduction would be 50 percent. It takes a prepared mind to realize that one learns nothing from relative values without first knowing the absolute values. It also takes a prepared mind to realize that when the difference in absolute values is trivial, the assertion that the difference is "statistically significant" does not mean that the difference is clinically significant. It only speaks to whether the difference is likely to occur by chance; if the trivial difference is deemed unlikely to occur by chance alone (that is, it is statistically significant), it is still a trivial difference that is clinically meaningless. It may be improbable because of any one of a number of unmeasured reasons, as we discussed above. One should have no confidence that it reflects anything we know or care about and no confidence that it will reproduce.

These considerations about relative risks, odds ratios, and other ratios are well known to epidemiologists, statisticians, clinical investigators, and nearly everyone else who is involved in clinical research. But you wouldn't know that from reading the scientific literature, even the premier journals. Ratio measures are always very accessible, while absolute values are often hidden in the text if not excluded.[32] Furthermore, there is a disconcerting tendency to present the relative risks and odds ratios in abstracts, often with the level of statistical significance but seldom with the absolute values.[33] Abstracts are summaries published up front in the scientific papers. Too often, the abstract is all that is read. Furthermore, there are many collections of abstracts designed to give the readership a heads-up on publications with the assumption that a serious reader will pursue the complete article. In fact, it is far more likely that abstracts are read without bothering to run down the rest of the article. Most authors and all involved in marketing are well aware of the powerful role of the abstract; some authors and all involved in marketing are also well aware that most of us do not have a prepared mind when it comes to analyzing the science that speaks to our health. We are easily scammed by ratio measures such as relative risk reduction. While scientific journals have gone to lengths to recognize issues of authorship, conflict of interest, and the structure of abstracts, attention to the use of ratio measures has not been emphasized. One might hope that the medical readership in general and scientific peers in particular might be a match for ratio measures. Asking other interested parties to assume responsibility for interpreting derivative data is asking a lot, however, and there are many interested parties, including the press.

Because of the demanding and specialized nature of the medical and scientific literature, a specialty in journalism — medical journalism — has come into being. The Association of Health Care Journalists, founded in 1997 and based at the University of Missouri School of Journalism, has more than 1,000 members. From the beginning, the association did not shy away from recognizing the moral hazards inherent in translating "health" news to the public. Today, health journalism is more beleaguered than most other specialties by the financial crunch that faces the entire Fourth Estate. Thanks to downsizing, there are fewer health journalists, and fewer yet who are not asked to cover additional aspects of the news. One fallback available to editors in such a circumstance is to purchase health coverage from leading journalists in the employ of other outlets. We have grown accustomed to this when it comes to finance, politics, sports, and international coverage.

But health reporting has access to another source, one that is particularly appealing given its packaging and low cost. This source hides behind the euphemism "Health Communications." We are bombarded by announcements and pronouncements from medical centers and even medical practices. Many tout the opening of a new building, or the offering of a new procedure, or a world-class expertise that outshines all others. These announcements and pronouncements are the product of a formal department in the institution that often bears the moniker "Public

Affairs" or even "Public Affairs and Marketing Office," as is the case for my own UNC Hospitals. The departmental budget is often liberal and part of the "overhead" of health care in our country. We all pay for these activities as part of our health-care premiums. Staffing these departments are people highly skilled in communicating to the public with backgrounds in marketing, public relations, or, increasingly, health journalism. Working in institutional "health communications" is all too often the soft landing for unemployed health journalists. Hence, the pronouncements and announcements are often put forth in compelling medicalese and in the glossiest of multimedia formats. There are websites that serve as the platform for this activity.

A recent analysis of the press releases by academic medical centers casts all this activity in an unflattering light.[34] This analysis was a demanding exercise undertaken by investigators funded by the National Cancer Institute. Academic medical centers issued an average of nearly fifty press releases annually. Nearly half pertained to research in animals that was almost always cast as relevant to human health. Of the releases about primary human research, very few were describing studies that would pass muster as high quality; far more described findings that were preliminary at best. Most neglected to emphasize cautions regarding interpreting such studies. Clearly, academic medical centers are wont to promote research that has uncertain relevance to human health. Nothing makes as much of a splash as the pronouncement of a 50 percent reduction or more in some untoward outcome. The audience has to learn to ask whether this 50 percent reduction is a difference of 60 out of 100 untreated versus 30 out of 100 treated, or 6 out of 10,000 versus 3 out of 10,000. The audience also has to learn how to demand honesty.

Screening for Cervical Cancer

In 1928 Dr. Georgios Nicholas Papanikolao, a Greek immigrant working at Cornell Medical School, reported that uterine cancer can be diagnosed if one studies the cells in vaginal secretions. The observation was largely ignored until 1943, the year Papanikolao and Herbert Traut published *Diagnosis of Uterine Cancer by the Vaginal Smear*, in which they detailed the normal and abnormal cells they saw under the microscope in the vaginal secretions of over 3,000 women. By the time Papanikolao published *The Atlas of Exfoliative Cytology* in 1954, the "Pap Test" was an established screening test around the world and cytopathology was an established discipline in clinical pathology. Over the next fifty years, much effort was expended to standardize the test and establish its specificity and sensitivity. As a consequence, we have learned much about uterine cancer and benefited great numbers of woman whose cancers were detected and removed before they had spread. More recent efforts have been directed at fine-tuning and are not without controversy. Unlike screening mammography, neither the fine-tuning nor the controversy has captured the public attention. Perhaps this relates to the fact that the Pap Test, unlike mammography, is a pretty good screening test for cancer of the cervix. It is not as good for detecting the cells of cancer inside the uterus, nor is it particularly useful in young, sexually active women who are at greatest risk of active infection with Human Papillomavirus (HPV), which can cause cervical cells in the secretions to look quite abnormal. As the active infection subsides, the cells return to their normal appearance, though HPV leaves a risk of future cervical cancer in its wake.

The Pap Test is a screening test; if positive, something else must be done to make or exclude the diagnosis of cervical cancer. Sometimes HPV is sought by DNA analysis, in which case the positive Pap Test in an older woman is more likely to reflect cancer than acute infection. Usually, a positive Pap Test results in the biopsy of anything that looks suspicious on direct inspection of the cervix during a pelvic examination. The biopsy is examined under the microscope and graded as to the degree to which the cells of the cervix appear abnormal. Minor degrees of abnormality are dismissed as likely to reflect HPV or other insults. When the cells are graded CIN 3, the lesion is considered precancerous. CIN is the acronym for Cervical Intraepithelial (in the lining cells) Neoplasia (abnormal cell growth). CIN 3 is likely to progress to invasive cancer, although the time from developing CIN 3 to developing invasive disease is about a decade (the dwell time).

So we have a reasonably sensitive screening test, a reasonable way to validate a positive (biopsy), a predictable natural history with plenty of time to intervene, and a cure (hysterectomy). There is still room to improve the specificity, sensitivity, and reliability of the Pap Test and the biopsy. But it is good enough to revisit the recommendations for cervical-cancer screening; many an august organization has felt compelled to do so repeatedly. In late 2009, the American College of Obstetricians and Gynecologists (ACOG) produced their latest iteration.[35] Given the state of screening and the dwell time, annual screening was not necessary. For women older than thirty and younger than sixty-five to seventy, screening every three years should be adequate. For women older yet who had repeatedly negative screening tests in the past, further routine screening was discouraged. It was felt that the inconvenience of the screening and of the biopsy of lesions that were unlikely to progress to invasiveness in their lifetime could not be justified.[36]

These recommendations rest easy in the United States. They are echoed by the American Cancer Society and the USPSTF and have engendered little push-back. Concerns have been raised about older women who continue to have multiple sexual partners and therefore possible exposure to oncogenic HPV infections.[37] There is even concern that by discontinuing screening, aging woman will have less reason to see a doctor periodically. This may be more important for the gynecologist and primary-care physician than for the patient, as there is very little to be gained by examinations that are not symptom driven. The debate over discontinuing cervical-cancer screening has quieted down in the United States for the moment, but not in Europe. The argument relates to the observation that while cervical cancer is less common in the older woman, it may be more aggressive.[38]

As is true for most countries with national health-insurance schemes, it is possible to use administrative data to inform this debate over stopping screening. Investigators in the Netherlands followed two groups of women for ten years after their third negative Pap Test: nearly 220,000 women aged forty-five to fifty-four and 445,000 aged thirty to forty-four. The incidence of cervical cancer did not differ in the two groups. Based on this, the Dutch concluded that age is not a good discriminative factor for early cessation of cervical-cancer screening. Yes, but this is age less than sixty-five, and no one is recommending cessation of screening under age sixty-five, just decreased frequency.

Realize that by screening 10,000 women between ages forty-five and fifty-five for a decade, the Dutch detected only four cases. Without screening, four women out of 10,000 would have died of cervical cancer before age sixty-five. Why, you might appropriately ask, am I cutting slack for screening for cervical cancer when I treated mammography harshly, even though mammographic screening of this same cohort might spare seven of these women death from breast cancer before age sixty-five? Good question. It's not because of the inconvenience of unnecessary biopsies; both screening mammography and Pap Tests increase the likelihood of "negative" biopsies. There are several reasons I am cutting the Pap Test slack. First, screening for cervical cancer has little risk of overtreatment. Second, there is no "cervical awareness" comparable to "breast awareness" that operates in the diagnostic limb to increase the likelihood that cervical cancer will be detected early without screening. Aside from vaginal blood spotting, there are few putative "early signs" of cervical cancer. Although mammographic screening *might* spare seven of these women death from breast cancer, diagnostics alone will do nearly as well, if not as well, without the risks of overtreatment thanks to "breast awareness." Finally, cervical cancer has a relatively homogeneous biology with a predictably long dwell time, so that early detection by screening can work. Breast cancers have heterogeneous biologies, including cancers with short dwell times that thwart early detection.

So I think the ACOG guidelines for screening for cervical cancer are defensible. Since I am not convinced that women older than sixty-five need routine gynecologic examinations for any other reason, and given the dwell time of cervical cancer, I would think that the ritual of the stirrups should be a rapidly dimming unpleasant memory for any woman over sixty-five who had a history of repeated negative Pap Tests.

Screening for Prostate Cancer

Prostates do not age gracefully. In young men, this is a walnut-sized bundle of glandular tissue encircling the urethra as it leaves the bladder. The glands are tightly stacked and curl their way into conduits that merge with the two ejaculatory ducts so that the prostatic secretions can mix with seminal fluid and sperm during ejaculation to accomplish some mysterious end that largely eludes scientific enquiry to this day. Several of the constituents of the prostatic secretions are relatively unique to this fluid. One, the protein prostate-specific antigen (PSA), is made exclusively by the glandular cells of the prostate. We have no idea what this substance is doing in the secretions, but there's a lot of it. However, the prostate's glandular elements are sloppy in making PSA; a small amount finds its way into the bloodstream, where it is fodder for the "PSA Test." If the gland is traumatized by a doctor's examining finger, or sitting on a bicycle seat, or an infection, or whatever else, more PSA is forced into the bloodstream. Furthermore, the more glandular cells there are, the more PSA that is leaked into the bloodstream.

As is true of nearly every tissue in the body, the glandular cells die a natural death to be replaced by neophytes without compromising the integrity of the gland. This normal turnover proceeds in a highly organized fashion with predictable periodicity in early manhood. By midlife, the programming for turnover loses discipline. Glands form that have no connections; glandular cells heap up, creating lumpy nodules; and the entire mass of glandular elements increases. Not long after midlife, all prostates are enlarged and nodular, so-called Benign Prostatic Hypertrophy (BPH). Often these nodules compress the urethra as it traverses through the prostate and interfere with urination, sometimes in ways that are troublesome or worse. (We will discuss this further in chapters 5 and 6.)

The disorganized turnover of the glandular cells is more than an issue in the architecture of the aging prostate. These cells have lost some of the biology that had determined their organizational capacity. However, the cells look normal under the microscope, and while they are capable of heaping up, they stay within the boundaries of the glandular elements. Some cells lose more of the normal biology and look abnormal under the microscope. If they still do not violate the territorial boundaries of the glandular element, this is analogous to "ductal carcinoma in situ," the infamous DCIS so common in the aging female breast. However, if they violate the boundaries of the glandular element and take up residence in the tissue between the glands, they become prostate cancer. These abnormal glandular cells tend to leak more PSA into the bloodstream than normal cells, even when they are still confined to the prostate gland. Once prostate cancer cells violate the capsule of the prostate, even more PSA gets into the blood.

By age sixty, every man should assume he has prostate cancer. If we were to examine their prostates thoroughly under the microscope, we'd find a focus or more of prostate cancer in the vast majority of men this age. Most of the time, it would be "early-stage" cancer, where the cells do not look too abnormal and have not ventured forth much at all. The five-year survival rate from such early-stage prostate cancer approaches 100 percent.[39] Obviously, nearly all men die with prostate cancer but very few from prostate cancer, and these nearly always late in life. Of those who die from prostate cancer, most would have died about the same time from something else (usually heart disease) had prostate cancer not been preemptive. However, there are a few who die from prostate cancer before their time, a dying that is prolonged and painful. The challenge is to somehow identify these unfortunate few men who are destined to die from prostate cancer before the cancer has progressed beyond the confines of their prostate. For these few men, and only these few, removal or otherwise destroying the prostate with some form of radiation spares them death before their time. All the others will never know they have prostate cancer because they will die from something else long before their prostate cancer is symptomatic. To treat all the others is the essence of "overdiagnosis" and "overtreatment."[40]

When I was a medical student, we were taught that a digital rectal examination was a necessary part of the routine physical examination for two reasons. First, one might palpate a rectal carcinoma, or at least get a stool sample to test for occult blood that might indicate that colorectal cancer was lurking. The second reason was to palpate the prostate, looking for ominous nodules. We now know that we were led astray: there is little if any utility to the digital rectal examination (DRE) or, for that matter, the routine physical examination, though both are still common practices. Colorectal cancer is the next topic. But the specificity of the DRE of the prostate is terrible because so many lumps and bumps represent nothing more than the aging process, or BPH. Even a finger of faith tainted by hubris can't reliably discern the occasional evil bump from all the rest. Early prostate cancer was a will-o'-the-wisp until two "advances" dragged the prostate out of hiding into the bright light of medicalization.

The first advance was a surgical advance that moved prostatectomy (surgical removal of the prostate) out of the annals of heroic surgical violence, where radical prostatectomy had resided next to radical mastectomy. Radical prostatectomy had long recovery times, many postoperative complications, and frequent long-term adverse consequences. The newer procedure was far less horrific—though no walk in the park. The second advance was the addition of the PSA to the DRE as a screening test. A positive PSA was to be followed by needle biopsy or biopsies, and a positive biopsy by a more limited and less morbid prostatectomy. This algorithm took foothold in the male conscience just as screening mammography did to women. PSA screening increased dramatically within a decade of its introduction in 1988.[41] By 2008 most men over fifty had had a PSA,[42] and so had nearly all male urologists and most primary-care physicians.[43] Of course, the detection rate of prostate cancer paralleled the increase in screening: the 20 percent likelihood of a positive PSA with repeated screening subsequently begot a 25 percent positive biopsy, which further begot a prostatectomy for an ever-increasing number of men.

The grumbling started over a decade ago.[44] Were we perpetrating overdiagnosis and overtreatment on the prostate similar to what we were doing to the female breast? A science was accumulating to suggest as much, strongly to my way of thinking. But as is true for screening mammography, those who were students of the science remained uncertain, and those who were committed to and involved in the screening algorithm pushed back. In 2008 the USPSTF felt that the evidence was insufficient to assess the balance of benefits and harms of screening for prostate cancer before age seventy-five, but there was enough evidence to call for halting screening after seventy-five.[45] In April 2009 the American Urological Association[46] pushed back by updating and confirming its "best practices" policy regarding screening for prostate cancer:

> The American Urological Association (AUA) and the AUA Foundation believe that early detection of and risk assessment for prostate cancer should be offered to asymptomatic men 40 years of age or older who have a life expectancy of at least 10 years. Men who wish to be screened should have both a prostate-specific antigen (PSA) test and a digital rectal exam (DRE). The decision to proceed to prostate biopsy should be based not only on PSA and DRE results, but should take into account multiple factors including free and total PSA, patient age, PSA velocity, PSA density, family history, ethnicity, prior biopsy history and comorbidities. The AUA strongly supports informed consent before screening is undertaken and the option of active surveillance, in lieu of immediate treatment, for certain men found to have prostate cancer.

Clearly, the AUA leans toward stamping out prostate cancer at all cost. "Active surveillance" is not defined but implies repeated PSAs and biopsies while coping with the knowledge that one's prostate is a time bomb. At the same time the AUA was advising screening from age forty, the American Cancer Society advocated annual screening after age fifty "after discussing risks and benefits with patients," and the American Academy of Family Physicians and the American College of Physicians echoed the USPSTF.[47] What's a fellow to do?

As was true for screening mammography, the controversy relating to the rational approach to prostate cancer did nothing to stay the hand of those who were involved in doing biopsies and committed to cure at all cost. PSA screening is common practice. Prominent men have trumpeted their triumph over cancer for the print and broadcast media. Malpractice suits have been won by men with prostate cancer who had not been offered PSA screening. Every therapeutic skirmish in the "War on Cancer" has captured the attention of the press and the people, including the battle of the prostate. Science has been silenced by the anecdotes of the survivors and by the residual uncertainty.

Truth be told, there is very little residual uncertainty in the scientific community. There is no doubt that PSA screening is a very flawed approach to sparing men death before their time from prostate cancer; few if any were spared, and many paid an awful personal price for the attempt. Some were driven to suicide by the diagnosis,[48] and nearly all suffered major compromises in their quality of life, regardless of how they were "cured."[49] Nonetheless, screening PSA had a life of its own until March 2009, a landmark for the prostate. Several very large, long-term randomized controlled trials of screening versus diagnostics that were begun in the 1990s were coming of age. In 2009 the results of two were published. The American trial (PLCO is its acronym) randomized some 75,000 men[50] to routine PSA/DRE screening or "usual care"; about half in "usual care" opted for a PSA at least once. The European trial (ERSPC) randomized 160,000 men between the ages of fifty-five and sixty-nine to routine screening or "usual care."[51]

PLCO conclusions: "After 7 to 10 years of follow-up, the rate of death from prostate cancer was very low and did not differ significantly between the two study groups."

ERSPC conclusions: "PSA-based screening reduced the rate of death from prostate cancer by 20 percent but was associated with a high risk of overdiagnosis."

As I said before, it requires a prepared mind to recognize the sophistry of offering relative risk reduction without knowing the absolute risk reduction. Both trials are in the vaunted *New England Journal of Medicine*, and these conclusions are in the abstracts. The truth behind the ERSPC abstract is as follows.

After nine years, the prostate cancer mortality was 0.29 percent in the screened group and 0.36 percent in the "usual care" group—a relative risk reduction of 20 percent, which was statistically significant. In other words, if you screen 1,400 men for nine years, screening would cause you to treat forty-eight additional men for cancer but avert death from prostate cancer in only one of them. That is certainly a lot of overdiagnosis and overtreatment for a tenuous benefit in the European trial that eluded detection in the American trial. But it is not enough for closure on the saga of the PSA. Methodologists can always find "what ifs?" in any such enormous trial. What if the men who were not invited for screening were not allowed to be screened by their own physicians? Many were in both trials, particularly in the PLCO, which "contaminates" the control group. What if African Americans were better represented in the PLCO? What if they were a tiny minority? What if . . . ?

Furthermore, the urologists are not willing to give up without a battle. The AUA statement displayed above was formulated in response to the publication of these trials. The USPSTF statement referred to above was formulated before the trials were published. A revised statement is about to appear. We can easily foretell its thrust.

To me, these trials demonstrate an unconscionable amount of over-diagnosis and overtreatment for such a tenuous benefit. I have never let anyone check my PSA based on earlier data. As for a DRE, pshaw. Now you, too, are fully informed.

As was true for screening mammography, there is nothing inherently wrong with the notion of screening. It's the test that stinks. Furthermore, there is no way to tweak the PSA as currently done and improve its util-ity.[52] I'd argue that we should stop screening for prostate cancer until we have a clinically relevant prognostic marker.[53]

Colorectal Cancer

I suspect that at this point, the reader could write this section. How do we avoid badgering all those people who are not at risk of dying from colorec-tal cancer and still identify the few who can be spared death before their time if their colorectal cancer is removed early enough? "Colonoscopy," you are primed to respond. After all, it should be possible to directly visu-alize the early lesion, prove its malignant nature by biopsy, and remove it.

It's not that simple in practice.

The provincewide experience in Ontario is an object lesson.[54] About 10,000 people aged fifty-two to ninety who were diagnosed with colo-rectal cancer between 1996 and 2001 had died of colorectal cancer by the end of 2003. These were compared to five people matched by age, sex, geographic location, and socioeconomic status that did not die from colo-rectal cancer. This is called a case-control study. About 700 case patients (7 percent) and 5,000 controls (10 percent) had undergone colonoscopy. Since the case patients were less likely to have undergone colonoscopy, colonoscopy might be useful for thwarting death from colon cancer. How-ever, when the difference was examined more closely, the only difference was in the likelihood of dying from colon cancer that had started in the left, or distal, half of the colon. There was no difference in the likelihood of death from cancer of the right half of the colon. The left half of the colon is the half closest to the anus. Would screening accomplish as much if only the left half of the colon was screened? This is not a facetious question.

Colonoscopy involves inserting a tube the length of the colon. One would not need colonoscopy to visualize just the left half of the colon. There is a shorter tube, a flexible sigmoidoscope, that would suffice. This is not a trivial distinction. Flexible sigmoidoscopy is easier on the patient and technically less demanding of the examiner. It requires no sedation, far less compulsive bowel preparation with laxatives, less time to do and therefore less patient time away from normal activities, and much less expense. It is also less dangerous: the purging and sedation for colonoscopy are not well tolerated by all older patients, particularly those with multiple diseases. Colonoscopy and sigmoidoscopy are two forms of endoscopy, which is the general term for looking inside any hollow organ but is usually applied to the gut. Both colonoscopy and sigmoidoscopy permit the endoscopist to biopsy growths and remove polyps. Biopsy is not without risk for complications, particularly in the elderly.[55] Major complications occur in as many as one or two patients out of every 1,000 who are endoscoped.[56]

There are several possible explanations for the observation that screening is more effective on the left half than on the right half of the colon. It is possible that death from right-side colon cancers would have been reduced in Ontario if those performing the colonoscopies were more skillful. Skillfulness matters. Another study from Ontario suggests that gastroenterologists miss fewer cancers than other physicians performing colonoscopy.[57] Detection rates vary by endoscopist — even when the endoscopist is a gastroenterologist — particularly as a function of how much time is taken exploring the colon.[58] While the case-control observations from Ontario suggest flexible sigmoidoscopy would do as well for screening as colonoscopy, case-control studies are far less definitive than randomized controlled trials. Randomized controlled trials comparing flexible sigmoidoscopy with colonoscopy are under way but will not conclude for many years.[59]

However, several randomized controlled trials comparing flexible sigmoidoscopy with usual care are nearing completion. Two were recently published. In one, the Norwegian Colorectal Cancer Prevention Trial,[60] nearly 56,000 people aged fifty-five to sixty-four were randomized to usual care (diagnostics) or once-only flexible sigmoidoscopy. Over the course of seven years of observation, there was no statistically significant difference in the incidence of colorectal cancer diagnosis or colorectal cancer mortality between the groups. Could it be that screening the colon, right or left, is a waste of time? Could it be that diagnostic programs driven by symptoms, or the incidental finding of anemia or blood hiding in the stool, work as well (or as poorly)? There is the suggestion that when this cohort is followed out for more years, the difference might be a bit more compelling and the advice for a single screening sigmoidoscopy on firmer footing.[61] But any advantage imparted to screening is likely to be quite small. The second study, a UK randomized controlled trial of once-only flexible sigmoidoscopy, makes this point.[62] Over 170,000 people between fifty-five and sixty-four years of age were randomized between 1994 and 1999 to sigmoidoscopy or not and followed ever since. There may be a slight reduction in death from colon cancer; the Number Needed to Treat (NNT) is calculated at nearly 500, but it's far from a robust effect.

Nonetheless, no one, including me, is advocating an end to screening by endoscopy for colorectal cancer. It is clear that if the screening by colonoscopy is negative at around age sixty, there is no reason for a follow-up for at least five years[63] — if not ten years, according to some guidelines, and never to my way of thinking. If screening by flexible sigmoidoscopy is as effective or nearly as effective, perhaps one negative flexible sigmoidoscopy sometime between age fifty-five and sixty-four is the best we can do in terms of screening to decrease the likelihood that we will die from colorectal cancer. That was my informed personal decision several years ago, even before the data were as compelling as they are today. I will not return for another endoscopy unless I have a concerning symptom.

I realize that I have now caused most readers to suffer cognitive dissonance. Most are hearing quite different advice from their physicians and others, and many have followed different advice. Many have been told their screening test was not negative because polyps were found and removed, and therefore they require surveillance with some frequency. Some are so advised, even when nothing is seen, in order to "play it safe." There are even dueling guidelines, published in 2008.[64] These guidelines pertain to "average-risk persons." There are high-risk persons who should be screened by colonoscopy early and repeatedly, such as people with a first-degree relative who developed colorectal cancer before age fifty and patients with ulcerative colitis or Crohn's colitis. For "average-risk persons," there are screening guidelines promulgated by the USPSTF and the "joint guidelines" drafted under the imprimaturs of the American Cancer Society, the U.S. Multisociety Task Force on Colorectal Cancer, and the American College of Radiology. It is worth our while to examine the process of drafting such guidelines as well as the guidelines themselves.

U.S. PREVENTIVE SERVICES TASK FORCE GUIDELINES

The USPSTF was first convened by the U.S. Public Health Service in 1984, and since 1998 it has been sponsored by the Agency for Healthcare Research and Quality (AHRQ), which is tucked into the Medicare administration.[65] The "task force" itself is an independent panel of private-sector experts in prevention and primary care. The USPSTF conducts rigorous, impartial assessments of the scientific evidence for the effectiveness of a broad range of clinical preventive services, including screening, counseling, and preventive medications. The USPSTF recommendation statements present health-care providers with information about the evidence behind each recommendation, allowing clinicians to make informed decisions about implementation.

The collecting and sorting of the evidence on particular topics is a monumental task. For this purpose, the USPSTF is supported by Evidence-based Practice Centers (EPCs). Under contract to AHRQ, each EPC conducts systematic reviews of the evidence on specific topics in clinical prevention. The USPSTF considers the systematic reviews, estimates the magnitude of benefits and harms for each preventive service, reaches consensus about the net benefit for each preventive service, and issues a recommendation.[66] The task force grades the strength of the evidence from A (strongly recommends), B (recommends), C (no recommendation for or against), D (recommends against), or I (insufficient evidence to recommend for or against).

Accordingly, the USPSTF commissioned an EPC to undertake a focused systematic review of the key questions relating to screening for colorectal cancer.[67] In addition, the USPSTF commissioned researchers affiliated with the National Cancer Institute to undertake a mathematical analysis comparing the utilities of various screening strategies and the age at which screening should start or stop.[68]

THE AMERICAN CANCER SOCIETY–U.S.
MULTI-SOCIETY TASK FORCE GUIDELINES

The American Cancer Society–U.S. Multi-Society Task Force (ACS-MSTF) published their guidelines[69] shortly before the USPSTF. The ACS-MSTF approached their task differently from the USPSTF. They did not undertake a systematic review of the literature or a decision analysis. The USPSTF and EPC staff is heavily weighted toward methodologists who are students of screening as a general clinical methodology. In contrast, the membership in the ACS-MSTF is heavily weighted toward specialists involved in various aspects of the diagnosis and management of colorectal cancer, for whom clinical experience and clinical judgment were considered powerful inputs into constructing their guidelines. For the ACS-MSTF, the goal of screening was not to diagnose colorectal cancer but to prevent it. Therefore, their focus was the identification and removal of the earliest of precancerous lesions, the polyp. Polyps are like grapes on a stalk where the grape is a collection of disorganized glandular elements comprised of cells that do not look abnormal under the microscope. It's the gut's answer to the prostatic nodules of BPH. These polyps are common and lend themselves to ready removal at the time of endoscopy by snaring the stalk and cutting it. And they are precancerous . . . barely so. The dwell time is measured in many years, if not decades. Yet, endoscopists love to snare them and are compensated for doing so. Patients come away with the belief that they have been unburdened of precancerous polyps for now, but that they have the propensity to make more precancerous lesions. Because of the focus on finding polyps, the ACS-MSTF constructed guidelines that differ from the USPSTF's, but not dramatically. The only dramatic difference is that the USPSTF advises against screening after age seventy-five.

The difference is more in perspective than in the details. This is reflected in a lengthy discussion of screening for colorectal cancer in the influential *New England Journal of Medicine* by David A. Lieberman,[70] who cochaired the ACS-MSTF. He advises that if there are no polyps on colonoscopy, repeat colonoscopy can be postponed ten years. Lieberman interprets the Ontario case-control findings by warning that "colonoscopy may not reduce the risk of proximal colon cancer (right sided) unless the examination is complete and all polyps are removed." If a polyp is found, he recommends "colonoscopic surveillance; interval for repeat colonoscopy depends on the pathological findings." Reminiscent of the argument about prostate cancer, gastroenterologists believe that larger polyps, particularly if the cells look abnormal, are more precancerous. There are major flaws in this reasoning,[71] not the least of which is the all-too-common propensity to ignore the issue of thwarting a colon cancer that would not be the cause of death. So ACS-MSTF is a boon for the colonoscopy industry despite a science that questions whether it is a boon for the patients.

The development of screening and treatment guidelines is an endeavor that nearly every medical specialty organization is undertaking. The reliance on "experts" on the ACS-MSTF is far more typical of this process than the USPSTF. Financial ties between guideline panel members and industry are common. In one study of forty-four guidelines, 87 percent of the authors had some form of industry tie[72]—funding for research, consulting fees, speakers' honoraria, and the like. More concerning is the intrinsically conflictual nature of asking experts to question their expertise and their practice styles. An analysis of the guidelines established by the American College of Cardiology and the American Heart Association demonstrates a shift over time toward opinion rather than higher quality evidence.[73] Subliminal or not, experts bring their biases and values to the table when constructing the practice guidelines that speak to their own practice styles and rewards.[74] To paraphrase George Bernard Shaw, you may need a hangman, but you don't ask the hangman who to hang.

Screening for colorectal cancer is running into the same block that stumbled mammography and PSA. For the person at "average risk," these are very blunt screening instruments. They are very likely to find disease in people for whom the finding is irrelevant and not particularly good at finding the disease that threatens the individual's life expectancy before it is too late. If we are to render these blunt instruments less blunt, we need to be able to find those individuals hiding among the "average risk" who are at high risk. That will require new insights leading to new markers of risk. If the markers are sufficiently specific and sensitive, they would become the new screening tests. Progress in the molecular basis of colorectal cancer offers promise.[75] However, testing the utility of new markers as markers for screening or diagnosis is as demanding as testing the utility of the old screening test. The difference is that we need not repeat all the old mistakes.

To Screen, or Not to Screen

As stated repeatedly, screening is seductive because it makes sense. It makes sense when one can do something about an important disease if it's caught early enough—any important disease and not just cancer. The rub relates to the sensitivity and specificity of the screening tests, as we've just learned. That's why in 2005 the USPSTF recommended against screening adults for glaucoma with the simple tools available in primary care. It's also why the USPSTF recommended against screening for asymptomatic carotid artery narrowing in the general adult population in 2007. The screening is simple and safe, starting with listening with a stethoscope for noise (bruit) in the carotid artery in the neck, which reflects obstruction to flow of blood to the brain. The degree of obstruction can be determined by a simple, noninvasive procedure that measures impedance to flow. However, some degree of obstruction is common, few go on to stroke and fewer still to a stroke on the noisy side, and surgical correction of the impedance offers no advantage to the asymptomatic patient. (In *Worried Sick*,[76] I discussed the marginal benefit that might accrue to the symptomatic patient.)

But the USPSTF is not infallible and not always prescient. Remember, it's a committee with "experts," each bringing preconceived notions to the task of valuing the results of the systematic reviews provided by the "experts" on the EPCs. None of the studies that go into each systematic review is perfect, ideal, and above criticism. No matter how much effort is expended in standardizing the fashion in which individual studies are weighted as to importance, personal bias cannot be eliminated. When faced with similar studies that come up with dissimilar results, it is human nature to be more inclined to forgive some methodological flaw in the study with the result that resonates with one's preconception. It is also small-group psychology that the expert with the more persuasive personality is more likely to carry the day. These are far more subtle perturbations of judgment than one finds in committees comprised of individuals with overt conflicts of interest. But they are no less important.

Let's revisit the example of screening for an abdominal aortic aneurism. The aorta is the main artery leaving the heart, passing through the chest and through the back of the abdomen into the pelvis, where it divides to enter the legs. Atherosclerosis is normal in the aging abdominal aorta. For some, particularly men and more particularly men who smoke, the process leads to more than a buildup of atherosclerotic plaque. It leads to damage to the wall of the aorta, so that it slowly expands and bulges out like a balloon, which is called an aneurism. When the bulge gets large enough, it can burst, leading to a catastrophic rapid death. Ultrasound examination of the abdomen can safely and comfortably define the size of the abdominal aorta, discern whether it is bulging, and determine the size of the aneurism, if there is one. Repairing the aorta used to be high-risk major surgery, but recently it has become possible to insert a type of stent, a tube through the bulge, thereby relieving the expanding pressure on the wall. Although the operative mortality and the likelihood of death from rupture are reduced by this procedure, overall survival is not changed;[77] these men have lots of vascular disease elsewhere just lying in wait. Since the procedure can decrease the likelihood of a catastrophic death by aneurismal rupture, why not screen all men by ultrasound? In 2005 the USPSTF could justify such a recommendation in men aged sixty-five to seventy-five who have ever smoked, a "Grade B" recommendation implying modest enthusiasm. The enthusiasm is limited because the endovascular repair (stent) is not perfect in effectiveness and not without risk. Besides, many men with large aneurisms die of something else, in which case repair is overtreatment. One of my patients, a renowned physician, and I had this discussion repeatedly as we watched his aneurism slowly expand year by year until he died of a stroke.[78]

There is more science to consider since the USPSTF came up with its "Grade B" recommendation for screening. A recent trial in Britain[79] randomized half of some 65,000 men aged sixty-five to seventy-four to ultrasound screening and followed the population for a decade. If an aneurism was detected, the ultrasound was repeated over time and repair offered if the bulge reached a certain size. Given the time frame, many of the repairs were by the older, risky operative procedure. There were 155 deaths related to an abdominal aortic aneurism in the screened group and twice that in the diagnostic group, for an absolute reduction in the risk of death of 0.4 percent. In other words, they screened about 30,000 men to find some 1,500 abdominal aortic aneurisms. They screened these 1,500 repeatedly and recommended repair if the aneurism grew rapidly or reached 5.5 cm. Despite screening, about 150 of these 1,500 men died of ruptured abdominal aortic aneurisms, half from aneurisms that were smaller than 5.5 cm. If these 1,500 had not been screened, about 300 would have died of ruptured aneurisms. Screening spared 150 deaths by ruptured aneurism. So the initial screening found the 5 percent of men aged sixty-five to seventy-four who were at risk of death from a ruptured aneurism. Subsequent screening spared 10 percent of at-risk men this mode of dying. That means you have to screen about 200 men aged sixty-five to seventy-four to spare one man death by ruptured aneurism, an NNT of 200. An NNT greater than 50 is barely compelling; I am inclined to dismiss an NNT of 200 as likely irreproducible and clinically irrelevant.

It is particularly disconcerting because so many who are screened and followed will have a preemptive repair that would have proved unnecessary since they would have died of something else before their aneurism ever ruptured. Nonetheless, the British investigators felt that this degree of salvage justified the cost of screening. At the same time, Danish investigators[80] reached the opposite conclusion based on a systematic review of the literature. Given the hugely greater costs in the United States, one can only guess at whether the USPSTF will come up with a "Grade B" when they revisit this topic. (Revisit the NNTs of mammographic screening in the discussion above now that you have this perspective.)

There is more to screening, and much more to screening after age sixty that is now a focus of the USPSTF.[81] It is not my intent to provide a compendium. My intent is to arm the reader with a perspective that will render screening beneficial to them. I am not alone in so doing.[82] Some more of this will rear up in the next chapter. But for now, you are a match for screening advice — whether from your physician, some august advisory panel, or full-page advertisements and billboards selling safe, noninvasive studies of your blood vessels, your chest, your heart, or your entire body in the hunt for some evil.

4

THE AGED WORKER

We discussed Figure 1 in chapter 1 in terms of its implications for the longevity of our species. It has much more to teach us. Realize how much longevity had improved prior to 1950, prior to the major medical advances that we now take for granted.

The incidence of death from bacterial infections such as tuberculosis and other bacterial pneumonias and typhoid had dropped dramatically before we had effective antibiotics. Deaths from measles, whooping cough, and diphtheria likewise decreased in number long before we had effective vaccination programs. An extraordinarily prescient medical scientist had called all these "artificial diseases" before the turn of the twentieth century.[1] Rudolf Virchow (1821–1902) was a pioneering Prussian pathologist who is in the medical pantheon for realizing that cells were the building blocks of all the body's organs. He should be twice represented in the pantheon for his other major contribution, the notion of "social medicine." Virchow argued that there were "artificial diseases" that "are attributes of society, products of false culture." He further argued that the secret to their treatment was in the "improvement of social conditions." Driven by these insights, Virchow was elected to the Reichstag, where he was influential in promoting public hygiene. Some of his other political agendas proved ignominious: he was anti-Darwinist, he rejected Semmelweiss's theory of antisepsis, and he advocated "craniometry." His notion of "artificial diseases" never took hold beyond public hygiene. We now know better. Sewers, clean water, and improved housing made a major difference in the incidence of deaths from infectious diseases in the first half of twentieth century. But the advancing longevity that occurred in the second half of the twentieth century is a consequence of the delayed onset of noninfectious "artificial diseases." It is a consequence of the evolution in the structure of society following World War II, so that the course of daily living became ever more salutary. Furthermore, there is a robust science that has parsed the elements of life course that are associated with this happy outcome, which when removed or absent render the outcomes far less happy. This science is termed "Social Epidemiology" in the United States and often "Life Course Epidemiology" in Britain. Some of the most important influences have been identified in the pursuit of gainful employment.

This topic requires consideration of several heavy-duty tropes that cut across many fields, including sociology, philosophy, and law. But it is a topic that has great moment for anyone over age sixty who is in the workforce. I am such a person, an aged worker. Furthermore, the fact that I am a scientist who has studied the aging of the workforce from a social and clinical perspective for decades does not mean I have avoided the challenges myself. To the contrary; I have personally experienced much of the gamut. The difference between me and many others in the aging workforce is that I was not blindsided by the shifting of the sands, and I am fortunate to have the wherewithal to be resilient. However, it's difficult to offer up an autobiographical narrative that is more a service to the reader than it is self-serving. In particular, there is a fine line between a discussion of overcoming personal challenges and gloating.

Ole Doc Hadler

It is no secret that American medicine has been in flux for several decades. The mantra is that America practices a brand of medicine that the rest of the world would emulate if they could afford to do so. But the cost of maintaining this putatively brilliant brand of medicine has been escalating at a pace that outstrips all measures of economic growth. The cost exceeded 17 percent of the Gross National Product before the recession of 2008, and its rate of escalation seems recession proof. The turmoil that is American medicine is a consequence of a series of attempts to rein in escalating costliness. There has been relatively little questioning of the value of the American brand of practice or of its leadership role in the world. Rather, all sorts of constraints and innovations have been attempted that are aimed at decreasing the cost of providing Americans with their cherished form of medical care.

I am aware of the financial goings-on, but these had nothing to do with my choosing to spend my life in medicine and were not even a minor focus of my career. I wanted to practice superlative medicine and teach others how to do so. By the new millennium, I had been on the faculty of the University of North Carolina for a little more than a quarter century. I was accomplished as a clinician, a clinical educator, and an investigator, and I was not lacking for recognition in all three arenas. After twenty-five-some-odd years on the faculty of one institution, I knew the players and the rules of the playing. I respected many for their accomplishments as physicians and scholars.

The problem was that I no longer recognized my workplace. North Carolina Memorial Hospital, "built for and by the people of the state of North Carolina," had morphed into UNC Hospitals. Our comfortable, familiar, and very intimate hospital was surrounded by construction sites and was gathering an enormous layer of administrators. The holes in the ground served a "we will build it, they will come" competitive agenda; the rationale for the tiers of administration was that this was necessary to render the new facilities profitable. In many ways, UNC was typical of the lemmings pursuing the American solution to the conundrum of reining in the cost without sacrificing the brand. Hospitals in neighboring towns were on the same track toward economy of scale by centralizing the most resource-demanding forms of health care. Major hospitals, particularly major academic hospitals, had to commandeer a great number of primary-care sites to funnel those most needy of the most profitable interventions to the citadel on the hill.

After 1970 administration and scholarship progressively became separate pathways in the academy. By 1990 I had little to do with the administration, and they returned the favor. The new millennium found me peacefully coexisting with the administration of what had been a medical school and now was a prototypical burgeoning American *academic health center* that still housed a medical school and clinical scholars but considered neither to be its primary raison d'être. I proudly declared myself a member of an "underground" clinical department and expended a great deal of effort collaborating with other members who considered excellence at the bedside the curriculum to be modeled for the next generation. I also spent a great deal of my year teaching general medicine to resident physicians and students and rheumatology to fellows in training and many a postgraduate assembly. It was the best of times and the worst of times.

The first shoe to drop came from Washington in 1996. It was a lawsuit brought by the U.S. Department of Justice against the University of Pennsylvania, and later the University of Virginia, for double-dipping on Medicare billings. The Department of Justice argued that since Medicare paid more per patient for a day in an academic hospital to cover the cost of trainee (resident) care, wasn't the billing for the supervision by faculty a form a double-dipping? The defense of excellence in educating the next generation was overshadowed by the need to maintain the double-income stream if the academic departments were to continue as profit centers. The fines were paid and a compromise fashioned. The faculty had to demonstrate that they cared for patients independent of the activities of the residents in order to bill independently. In fact, their presence on "work rounds" was no longer tolerated.

The second shoe to drop was New York State's Libby Zion Law in 1989. Libby Zion was an eighteen-year-old college student who died in New York Hospital under the care of resident physicians who were deemed negligent because they were overworked and overtired. The law set the precedent for limiting the number of consecutive hours resident physicians could be required to work. In 2003 the Accreditation Council for Graduate Medical Education adopted similar regulations for all American medical schools: residents could not work more than eighty hours per week or more than twenty-four consecutive hours. These regulations are currently under review since there is no evidence they influence patient outcomes.[2]

The third shoe to drop on the vaunted American system of bedside teaching was the Hospitalist Movement. After all, since the residents had to get home for their rest, let's hire postgraduate residents to substitute when the residents are resting in their beds.

All of this seems rational. Only the experienced clinicians knew the downsides. Neither local administrations nor legislators could imagine there were any, but demanding that experienced physicians earn their keep away from the trainees destroyed the American model of bedside teaching. No longer were Socratic interchanges and literature references commonplace. The name of the game became managing the patient's case as expeditiously as possible instead of understanding the patient and the patient's plight. Training program goals changed from camaraderie in the quest of clinical perfection to lonely residents trying to finish up and get out of the hospital. That became possible because "hospitalists" would cover. But hospitalists have no idea who they are seeing before they are called to see them. They depend on the hospital record, often an electronic record that offers absolutely no clue to the person in the bed—only the person's disease, which is often wrongly described. Electronic medical records sound like a great idea. However, they lend themselves to being form rather than substance. I am accustomed to seeing a cardiac exam recorded as "present" and historical notes repeatedly "cut and pasted."

To make matters worse, the tiers of administrators brought corporate jargon with them. Patients became "units of care" and physicians became "providers." Both categories were considered readily replaced. The enterprise was devoted to "throughput." It is the business model that made McDonald's a titan. Shouldn't it work for patients and hospitals?

It didn't. But that is not my thesis in this chapter. There I was, comfortable in my skin, proud of my skills as a teacher and clinician, appreciated by my peers—but considered an anachronism, an expensive throwback, by the administration. I was tenured and able to confront this sea change with considerable personal resources. I will tell you what I did at the end of the chapter. Let's examine the science that informs a decision such as I had to make, and let me ask you what you would do.

The Challenge to My Job Satisfaction in Context

The Bureau of Labor Statistics (BLS) is a comprehensive, ongoing resource for anyone interested in descriptive statistics and demographics for the U.S. workforce. The BLS traces its roots to the Bureau of Labor Act of 1884 and has been housed as an independent agency in the Department of Labor since 1913. It is charged with finding the "facts" that relate to labor economics and statistics and making such available to the government and any other interested party. The BLS provides fodder for labor economists and policy makers, whether they are part of the Congressional Budget Office, actuaries employed in insurance companies, or anyone else who needs to understand labor trends. Most of these people are employed as soothsayers. *Rethinking Aging* is not attempting to predict the future for the youth of today. We are examining the circumstance of those who are over sixty today in the United States and elsewhere in the resource-advantaged world. This chapter considers those over sixty who are gainfully employed. Hence our focus is on two generations: those born between 1925 and 1945 and those between 1945 and 1965. It is common to refer to the former as the "traditionalists" and the latter as the "boomers." Both participate in the workforce, where they are joined by

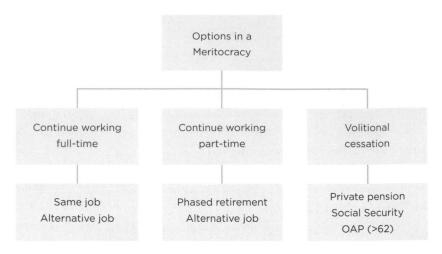

Figure 3. Options for the aged worker in a meritocracy.

members of "Generation X" (born between 1965 and 1980) and "Generation Y" (born between 1980 and 2000). The ramifications of the mix are far greater than chronological. Surveys document that these younger generations bring different attitudes to the workplace. They are less driven to climb the administrative ladder and far less likely to feel allegiance to their employer. Furthermore, each generation has its own sense of a "normal" balance between life at work and life outside work.

Negotiating this attitudinal mix is not the only challenge facing the employed boomers and traditionalists in the current economy. The architecture of work has changed. For example, many jobs are physically dispersed to "home offices" and sites around the world. The content of work—the demands of its tasks—has changed and continues to change rapidly, requiring flexibility in skills. Perhaps the most dramatic change is the contingent nature of employment. For the younger generations, downsizing, pink slipping, redundancy, and the like are facts of life in the workplace. For the boomers and traditionalists, these are counterintuitive happenstances, if not cataclysmic.

The boomers and traditionalists are not without personal resources on these shifting sands. They are endowed with whatever attributes of attitude, judgment, and flexibility they derive from experience. These attributes are the prerequisites for aging productively in the workplace, for becoming an *aged* worker rather than simply an *old* worker. The aged worker has achieved a station of comfort in life at work and in life outside of the workplace that working sustains and nurtures. "Aged" is not just a

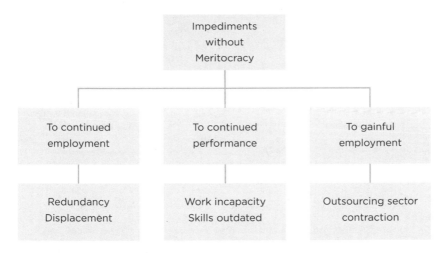

Figure 4. Impediments for the aged worker without a meritocracy.

chronological notion; it's a mindset. It denotes the self-confidence that derives from the acquisition of a competence that is valued. For the traditionalists, "aged" was predictable in a meritocracy. One worked to acquire skills and knowledge while expecting to be rewarded with job security and job autonomy. For the aged worker in a meritocracy, each passing year brought with it important choices.

The erosion of the meritocracy blindsided the traditionalists in the workforce, and they are now trying to regroup. These changes were far less of a surprise for the boomers; they have grown up with this erosion. Neither generation is comfortable with employers who invest less and less to garner their allegiance. The challenge to being successful demands more than performance; the challenge is to be able to invest oneself in the agenda of the employer in the absence of reciprocity. Generations X and Y contemplate a future with multiple jobs and therefore multiple transitions. For Generations X and Y, the menu in Figure 3 is an abstraction, even an anachronism. Little do they realize the mark on the quality of life its absence bodes when they are aged, if they ever arrive at aged (Figure 4). Traditionalists and boomers experience cognitive dissonance with such a tenuous station in life.

If this wasn't grief enough, we are living through an era where the "economy" causes many to try to maintain gainful employment longer than they had anticipated. The trend toward working longer in life was apparent before the recession of 2008 (Figure 5). The U.S. Census Bureau predicts that the number of workers over age fifty-five will escalate from

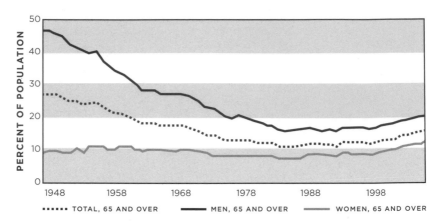

Figure 5. Labor force participation rate of workers age sixty-five and over, 1948–2007. The trend toward maintaining gainful employment after age sixty-five started to escalate before the recession of 2008. There is no doubt that the need to maintain gainful employment has been escalating ever since. We will learn before long whether the availability of employment is keeping pace and whether the employment options are sustaining. (Source: U.S. Bureau of Labor Statistics)

19 million in 2002 to 32 million by 2015, a prediction that requires all sorts of assumptions about the availability of jobs, the age that qualifies for retirement benefits, and the largesse of pensions. If correct, the percentage of the workforce over age fifty-five will escalate from 14 percent to 20 percent in this time frame.[3] Furthermore, many of these workers with career jobs will transition to self-employment.[4]

Clearly, the notion of the aged worker is a moving target at best and ephemeral at worst—and it always has been. A meritocracy is not evidence of innate altruism. To the contrary, the meritocracy that the traditionalist generation enjoyed is unique in history. Meritocracy resolves the innate conflict between "you butter my bread and I'll butter yours" and whatever tendencies the boss or owner has for extra dabs of butter. In the context of the workplace, meritocracy has always been market contingent. The boss valued the productive worker as long as the worker was productive to the benefit of the boss. That was as true of the landholder in an agrarian society as the factory owner in an industrialized society. The meritocracy of the last half of the twentieth century was highly enlightened, with rules of behavior on the part of the boss and the worker that were often negotiated transparently and even regulated by government. Some of the rules could be codified because the content of work in a manufacturing society is largely stereotypical and predictable; the worker produces so much, for which the worker is rewarded commensurately. The proviso "as long as the worker was productive" is the rub. In my last book, *Stabbed in the Back*,[5] I discuss the history of disability determination from the Elizabethan Poor Laws to the present. It's an uneven history, to say the least. The history of "old-age pensioning" is less uneven, in part because it commences in the twentieth century with a uniform template but, more important, because a worker's age, unlike his or her work capacity, is incontrovertible. Before turning our attention to "old-age pensions," we must examine what is known of life in the workplace for the aged worker.

Still Thriving at Work

Much of the information we have about life in the workforce, as well as outside of the workplace, speaks to what can and does go wrong. Information of this nature as it relates to the health of the aged worker will be examined in the next section. There is a need to understand what can go *right*, what can advantage the worker who persists in the workforce. The hints we have relate both to personal resilience and workplace factors. Do not assume that work, working, and working longer are intrinsically bad for you. Even in a less-industrialized but resource-advantaged country like Greece, for every five years longer someone in the general population stays employed, mortality decreases 10 percent.[6] Of course, there are many factors that can account for this and many subsets who are not advantaged by work, but "work" is a highly ambivalent four-letter word. Gainful employment can be salutary, or not. A century ago, the physical demands and physical exposures of tasks were influential in this regard, sometimes overwhelmingly so. Today, in any resource-advantaged country, the physical content of tasks has taken a backseat to contextual influences in the sociology of working.

Our current understanding of such contextual influences is rooted in the scholarship of David Émile Durkheim. Durkheim's ascension to the chair of pedagogy at the Sorbonne fin de siècle was circuitous. The scion of a long line of French rabbis, he chose a secular, academic path. Because his early interest in applying scientific principles to social issues (what we call social science) was anathema in the Cartesian tradition, he spent many of his student years in Leipzig. He returned to France to find that his bent toward socialism marginalized him in the academy of the Third Republic. He persevered and emerged as one of the fathers of modern sociology. Durkheim was fascinated with the way societies can survive despite ever-increasing heterogeneity. He developed notions of social cohesiveness and social capital. Social cohesiveness speaks to the connectedness among groups; social capital speaks to the norms of reciprocity and mutual aid. Because these "social facts" are forces in and of themselves, they are greater than the sum of the actions of individuals. Rather, these social facts can influence, even determine, the action of the individuals that comprise a societal grouping.

A century later, we have come to realize that these social facts are prime determinants of the longevity of any resource-advantaged societal grouping.[7] Some of the relationships are dramatic. In a classic state-by-state survey, the more the adults responded in the affirmative to the assertion that "most people would try to take advantage of you if they got the chance," the greater the death rate.[8] The association of measures of social capital with longevity parallels that with income inequality across the states. As is true for income inequality, there is also far less social capital in the American South than in the northern Midwest. Social capital is a normative construct, a feature of the group as a whole. It is the sum of many interpersonal dynamics, such as trust and social support. The latter has to do with the number and frequency of positive interpersonal relationships. Each of the components has an influence — often an easily measurable influence on the health of the participating individuals. All of these influences come together to form social capital, which, as said above, is a far greater influence on the health of the group than simply the sum of the interpersonal and personal factors.

Durkheim's realization of the important influence of social capital on the health of the group is a legacy that drives sociologists and some students of public health to this day. All sorts of populations and peoples have been viewed through this lens. Much of this work has been reductionistic; it is easier to probe for associations of components of social capital with the composition and dynamics of the group over time than to validate some composite measure of social capital. There are many associations that emerge in nearly all studies — socioeconomic status, education, health-adverse behaviors, violence, social support, injustice — and more that are associated with one another and with particular health outcomes. There are exceptions, such as in the emerging democracies of eastern Europe, where socioeconomic status and educational achievement are far less closely associated than in established democracies. There are also degrees of association between these factors that vary somewhat between populations. I discussed the relationship of social capital with longevity in the last chapter. Its importance as a determinant of the health of populations remains an interesting and productive line of investigation,[9] though inherently limited by the sluggish response of the social capital of community-based populations to perturbations in any of its component factors. When there is, such as in times of war, revolution, or coup d'état, the resulting chaos and realpolitik preclude data gathering.

I credit Robert Karasek and Töres Theorell[10] for realizing that the "workforce" offered a laboratory for studying social capital—a laboratory where the insights gained might be turned to the advantage of the workers. This notion was met with considerable resistance by ergonomists, industrial hygienists, occupational physicians, spine surgeons, and the workers' compensation industry, who were all wedded to the notion that excessive physical demands of tasks were the principal factors threatening the health of workers.[11] But with escalating zeal over the past several decades, investigators around the world have come to focus on the sociology of the workplace. As is true for community-based studies, this line of investigation has also been reductionistic. Furthermore, in common with most twentieth-century studies on occupational health and safety, the research is largely focused on the consequences of negative influences on social capital in the workplace. Many important insights have resulted, as will become clear in the following section of this chapter. What is less well represented in this literature is what can be done to enhance social capital in the workforce and whether doing so would prove salutary.

In order to study the influence of social capital on the health of a workforce, one needs an operational definition, something to measure. There is nothing straightforward about such a definition and no consensus in the literature.[12] There are social dimensions to the term, such as a sense of community, a feeling of integration, and the quality of interpersonal networks. There is also a capital dimension, the notion that a community takes a position in the marketplace. Two studies from Scandinavia are exemplary in attempting to parse influences of aspects of workplace social capital on the health of the workforce.

The Finnish Public Sector Study enrolled the municipal employees and hospital personnel of ten towns in 2000–2002, some 32,000 of the former and 16,000 of the latter. At baseline, these employees were questioned as to health-risk behaviors, diagnosis of depression and psychological distress, and many other personal factors. They also responded to a series of questions and statements designed to probe cognitive and structural components of social capital that have a moral dimension based on elements of trust and trustworthiness:[13]

1. "We have a 'we are together' attitude."
2. "People feel understood and accepted by each other."
3. "We can trust our supervisor."
4. "People in the work unit cooperate in order to help develop and apply new ideas."
5. "Do members of the work unit build on each other's ideas in order to achieve the best possible outcome?"
6. "Our supervisor treats us with kindness and consideration."
7. "Our supervisor shows concern for our rights as an employee."
8. "People keep each other informed about work-related issues in the work unit."

A follow-up questionnaire was administered three years later. Of the respondents who were not depressed at baseline, 5 percent had been started on antidepressant medication. Most were single women who had health-adverse behaviors and psychological distress. The presence of psychological distress at baseline was an important determinant of developing major depression. However, the risk of developing depression[14] and the likelihood of succumbing to health-adverse behaviors is attenuated by increasing social-capital behaviors in Finland as it is in the United States.[15] Furthermore, the effect of social capital is so robust that it is discerned for both a vertical and a horizontal component.[16] The former refers to relationships across institutionalized power gradients and the latter to relationships at the same hierarchical level. The more positive these relationships are, the less one's working life will contribute to the onset of a major depression.

There is a parallel study in Sweden that considers another dimension of social capital, one that emphasizes social contacts and participation in social networks. This aspect of social capital requires stability in demographics and attitudes. It is an aspect of social capital that is a double-edged sword; it is inherently exclusive, even to the extent of xenophobia. However, for those participating in the network, this aspect of social capital is long known to be salutary. A group of scientists in Malmö, under the direction of Martin Lindström,[17] recruited a cohort of over 10,000 workers aged forty-five to sixty-nine. They were assessed at baseline as to their perception of the psychosocial conditions at work and their level of social participation. Psychosocial conditions at work were defined according to a model[18] that probed the ratio of perceived control and decision latitude versus demands on the worker in terms of pace, intensity, and skillfulness. They were assessed a year later for degree of social participation during the year by a questionnaire as to participation in study groups, unions or other organizations, cultural or athletic activities, social gatherings, and so forth. Those people who described a favorable balance between work autonomy and task demands at baseline were more likely to have participated socially in the following year. They are also more likely to report that they are healthy and to live longer, if Swedes are like Danes.[19] The relationship between job satisfaction and self-assessment of physical and mental well-being is robust and generalizes widely across populations.[20] The degree to which self-reported health status and mortality correlates varies across populations, even across the United Kingdom.[21]

WORKING ON THIN ICE
Alone in my borrowed space,
Working for a boss who cannot listen,
Skills valued less, valueless;
Options . . . few, ephemeral:
My body hangs heavy on my frame.
What can set me free?[22]

The argument that inadequacies in social capital have health consequences in the general population is incontrovertible (see chapter 1). It is true that these inadequacies associate with such health-adverse behaviors as obesity and smoking.[23] But it is also true that health-adverse behaviors account for relatively little of the harm wreaked by compromised social capital.[24] The argument that inadequacies in social capital have health consequences in the working population, particularly for the aged worker, is also incontrovertible.

This does not mean that the compromise in social capital is the only challenge faced by the older worker. Elements of decrepitude are important, too. In the modern workplace, the aged worker may face challenges in terms of age-dependent physical impairments, particularly visual and auditory impairments.[25] This is not a trivial matter. While older workers are less likely to suffer violent, traumatic injuries than younger workers, they face more serious consequences.[26] There are several reasons for the decreased risk for traumatic injuries in older workers, including "survivor bias," in which those more prone to injury retire earlier from physically demanding tasks;[27] an older worker performing physically demanding tasks is more prone to seek disability retirement for the next backache;[28] and the "survivors" are advantaged by the degree to which experience mitigates any age-related impairments.[29]

However, continuing to perform customary tasks, even with increasing overtime, is not the principal challenge to maintaining employment.[30] The impediments for the aged worker lurk in the social capital, or lack thereof, of the particular workforce. There are multiple aspects of life in the workplace that correlate with burnout, absenteeism, disability retirement, and involuntary retirement; injustice,[31] bullying,[32] and hostile organizational structure[33] are examples that have emerged. Robyn Gershon's study is illustrative; she and her coworkers assessed the personal price that aging New York police officers are paying when they find their work stressful.[34] Work stress was assessed by probing feelings such as "I feel negative, futile, or depressed about work" and "My interest in doing fun activities is lowered because of my work" and by probing for situational stressors such as "There is good and effective cooperation between units" and "Promotions in the department are tied to ability and merit." The more stressful, the more likely the police officer was to "burn out," have chronic back pain, abuse alcohol, be depressed, or manifest inappropriately aggressive behavior.

The most dramatic experiments with social capital in the workplace have occurred when social capital is expunged by involuntary termination of employment, be it redundancy, downsizing, or the closing of the enterprise. Even the threat of downsizing can induce easily measured psychological distress.[35] The Finnish ten-town study discussed earlier offers an illustration of the magnitude of this assault on well-being. The municipal workforces of these ten towns were enrolled in a longitudinal study undertaken by the Finnish Institute of Occupational Health decades ago.

In the early 1990s, the Finnish economy tanked and unemployment surged to nearly 20 percent. The response of some but not all of these municipalities was to downsize their workforces. Just the specter of downsizing precipitated a dramatic increase in sickness absence, particularly among workers over age fifty.[36] Much of the sickness absence related to low back pain, which can be rendered less tolerable by such psychosocial challenges as job insecurity.[37] In fact, the cost of health care and disability pensioning was more than the monies saved in downsizing, even in a country with a very efficient national health-insurance scheme.[38] But the price paid by this workforce goes beyond their disabling backaches.

Within several years, the workers who were laid off were five times more likely to suffer a fatal heart attack than workers matched for age and gender employed in municipalities that did not downsize.[39] Furthermore, the remaining workers in the municipalities that downsized were at a lesser but measurable increased risk of a fatal heart attack.

The inescapable conclusion, based on the ten-town study and similar analyses elsewhere, is that having secure employment in favorable working conditions greatly reduces the risk of healthy people developing limiting and disabling illnesses.[40] Social capital is not to be taken lightly by anyone interested in the health of the workforce, if not the public at large. When it is tampered with, it is the older person who pays the price first.

"Flow" and Human Capital

When you reckon up the national wealth and begin to talk about imports and exports ... I have never seen a balance-sheet of that kind up to the present that did not omit the greatest asset of all, and that is the men, the women and the children of the land.[41]

Industrial psychologists speak of the personal impact of social capital as "flow," something akin to feeling comfortable in your skin. There will be good and bad days inside and outside of the workplace for all of us. But if, on balance, it seems worth it, then the career is fulfilling, the retirement deserved, and the life enjoyed longer until the inevitability of its ending. As we've discussed, workers who are disaffected or disavowed are more likely to experience affective disorders and more likely to succumb to health-adverse behaviors, including substance abuse. They are more likely to "burn out" and to have difficulty coping with other challenges at work or at home. For example, a disaffected worker is no more likely to experience an episode of low back pain or arm pain but is far more likely to find the pain intolerable. The resulting visits to physicians, sick leave, and workers' compensation claims for regional musculoskeletal "injuries" are the outward manifestation of the compromised coping ability that reflects compromised flow.[42] But all this pales in comparison to the most serious consequence associated with relentless dissatisfaction at work; namely, the disaffected worker does not live as long. Their longevity approaches that of the unemployed, who on average live five to seven years less than the gainfully employed in their birth cohort.

Social capital is the underpinning of flow, and flow the underpinning of productivity. This is what is meant by human capital. Workers are not machines. Adverse aspects of the psychosocial context of working, challenges of perceived or real illness, and resentment over the pay scale are all examples of negative influences on flow. Overtly or subliminally, such influences make it less likely that the worker will perform optimally. This is the notion of "presenteeism." Traditionally, health-related absence was calculated as a major indirect cost of doing business. It is now clear that health-related decreases in productivity while still at work are a greater indirect cost.[43] Low back pain provides a ready object lesson in the relationship between flow and presenteeism.[44] Presenteeism is the hidden cost of devaluing human capital.

There is no ready mechanism to assuage the assault on the "flow" of the aged worker as the modern economy transforms from the welfare state that nurtured the traditionalists and boomers to a form that satisfies the ongoing sea change described by Neil Gilbert, a social scientist at the University of California, Berkeley.

> To suggest that the welfare state as we knew it is being left behind somewhere along the path of institutional evolution does not signify the end of social welfare programs. . . . But the social policy environment in which they evolve will be constrained by a set of demographic and market conditions and informed by normative assumptions that are fundamentally different than those underlying the development of social welfare programs through the early 1980s. These structural conditions and social norms give rise to a new institutional framework that subordinates social welfare policies to economic considerations, such as the need for labor force flexibility, the opening of new markets for the private sector, the pressures of international competition, and the imposition of limits on deficit spending. Within this new framework, social welfare policies are increasingly being designed to enable more people to work and to enable the private sector to expand its sphere of activity.[45]

No doubt we are hell-bent on developing an "enabling state." No doubt the younger generations of workers can become accustomed to job mobility/insecurity, even gain skills that facilitate transitions. No doubt these generations of younger workers are destined to be the generations of older workers. But I doubt many among them will ever be aged workers. Furthermore, I have grave concerns as to whether many will know much "flow" in the workplace, let alone the longevity of their parents.

These doubts need strident voices as we construct the economy of the twenty-first century.

The value of social capital for the creation of human capital is a hard sell in an enabling state where productivity reigns supreme. It is also a hard sell for the well-being of the worker, given the entrenched beliefs of organized labor regarding the importance of the content of work despite the science establishing the greater importance of the context of working on the welfare of the worker. Nonetheless, I am optimistic that the importance of social capital will work its way into the common sense before long. I am not fearful that work and the workplace will transform into a New Age version of the brutal workplace scenario Jack London described in *People of the Abyss* (1902). Our communitarian ethic would not countenance such a direction. We are wedded to providing recourse for disability and for the contingencies of older age. Our approach to disability determination is flawed, as I detailed in *Stabbed in the Back*,[46] but not without redeeming and redeemable features. Our approach to "retirement" begs similar treatment.

Old-Age Retirement Pensions

Perhaps it is this specter that most haunts working men and women: the planned obsolescence of people that is of a piece with planned obsolescence of the things they make.[47]

In the early nineteenth century, it was a rare working man who "retired." Most expired long before such might be feasible. The elderly were not that old and were predominately widows dependent on their children for support. In the United States at fin de siècle, half the population had died by age fifty. This demographic changed little in the first half of the twentieth century (see Figure 1 in chapter 1). Faced with the aging workforce of that day, European states adapted a Prussian precedent to develop national insurance and annuity schemes to provide for the elderly as well as the infirm and disabled. Aside from workers' compensation insurance schemes, such legislation was mired in political debate in the United States.

The plight of the elderly, in particular, weighed heavily on the national ethic. In the Great Depression, that plight became more than unconscionable; it was an anger-engendering reproach. About half the elderly could not even sustain themselves. A physician, Dr. Francis Townsend, called for a monthly pension for every one over sixty to be paid for by a national sales tax with the stipulation that the pension must be spent rapidly. The idea was to kill two birds with one stone: improve the plight of the elderly while salving the Great Depression itself. There were organizations all over the country promoting the Townsend Plan and others promoting alternatives. As President Franklin D. Roosevelt described:

> Security was attained in the earlier days through the interdependence of members of families upon each other and of the families within a small community upon each other. The complexities of great communities and of organized industry make less real these simple means of security. Therefore, we are compelled to employ the active interest of the Nation as a whole through government in order to encourage a greater security for each individual who composes it. . . . This seeking for a greater measure of welfare and happiness does not indicate a change in values. It is rather a return to values lost in the course of our economic development and expansion.[48]

Neither the Townsend Plan nor Dr. Townsend were appealing to FDR. Rather, he favored a national old-age annuity fund, later called Social Security, matched by federal funds termed Old Age Assistance. FDR's vision was legislated in the Social Security Act, which passed Congress in August 1935. At the signing, FDR proclaimed: "We can never insure one hundred percent of the population against one hundred percent of the hazards and vicissitudes of life, but we have tried to frame a law which will give some measure of protection to the average citizen and to his family against the loss of a job and against poverty-ridden old age." The first pensions were disbursed in 1942 to anyone over sixty-five, prorated to one's earning history. The subsequent history of the Social Security Act is a battle as to the largesse of the pension program. Suffice it to say, subsistence in old age has never again been an issue for the workers of America, and, since the passage of Medicare thirty years later, neither have most forms of medical care. The challenges for the American worker relate to maintaining gainful employment until the age that qualifies for a Social Security pension and to come to grips with whether such a pension is adequate to sustain a satisfying life afterward. Both challenges are layered in psychosocial contingencies.

As stated above, part of "flow" is the knowledge that whenever the time is right, a comforting retirement awaits. Social Security may provide for such for some, but not for those who might wish to retire before sixty-two or those for whom Social Security alone would provide a lifestyle that is a shadow of what was enjoyed during years of employment. For these aged workers, pensions offer that promise. Early in their careers, pensions were assumed to be secure. Many were tied to the fortunes of the enterprise to which they had hitched their career wagon. No one assumes that pensions are inviolate any longer.

Peter Drucker was one of the giants of twentieth-century capitalism, a self-described "social ecologist." Drucker was to management what W. Edwards Deming was to quality initiatives and John Maynard Keynes to economics. Among his many contributions, Drucker understood the importance of human capital and the need to envision a corporation as a human community. Drucker realized that the notion of a pension tied to one's corporate home was only as secure as the ability of that corporation to grow in profitability. If not, the "dependency ratio" would put the pension at risk. Malcolm Gladwell revisited this notion in an elegant essay, "The Risk Pool," in the August 28, 2006, issue of the *New Yorker* magazine. As the corporation ages, a growing fraction of its productivity must serve the needs of the growing number of pensioners. This demands ever greater productivity and profitability. That requires inventiveness and facile leadership. Lacking either can be catastrophic for the pensioners of a mature corporation, if not for the employees. For example, by the mid-1990s, serving the benefits programs of current and retired employees required all of the profits of General Motors car and truck divisions; only the finance division was profitable. The more recent supplanting of employer-provided pensions to employee-owned and -managed, tax-deferred annuities moves the pension out from under the uncertainties of long-term corporate solvency to the vagaries of the financial markets. Social Security does not escape these considerations. As currently constituted, the tax burden of its provision will increase as the pensioner pool grows. Privatizing adds management overhead to the uncertainties of the financial markets.

The size and stability of pensions are critical to enjoying the Golden Years.

Meeting the Challenge to My Job Satisfaction

I promised I'd tell you what I did when faced with my Rubicon as an aged worker. It was a very painful time. With a feeling of great loss and personal pain, and some anger, I stated out loud that if I can't teach according to my conscience at the bedside at UNC Hospitals, I won't teach there at all. I still see many outpatients. And I still teach inpatient medicine as an invited visiting professor at institutions around the world. But it is painful to see the day-by-day activities at my institution and at others in the United States. It is so painful that I embarked on a path to teach America how/why its vaunted health-care system has lost its way and is now ethically bankrupt. *Rethinking Aging* is the fourth book in my attempt to do so.

I can only wish that other aged workers facing their Rubicon could choose to walk a different path and do so unscathed. Few are so fortunate. Most will pay a terrible personal price in terms of their sense of worth and their health. This is happening all too often. We all need to decry the current dialectic.

5

DECREPITUDE

It was the best of times, and then the worst, for Mrs. K.

Mrs. K. was a seventy-year-old woman enjoying her Golden Years. She actively participated in the life of her family and her community. She enjoyed robust good health and a vigorous lifestyle. She woke one morning feeling well, until she attempted to leave the bed. There was a sudden gnawing pain between her shoulder blades, which rapidly escalated in intensity when she attempted to rise up from the bed. She laid still, head elevated on the pillow, and was comfortable again. She was not breathless, but a deep breath reminded her that something was amiss, and another attempt at rising informed her forcefully. With great difficulty, she managed to toilette and dress, but then she found herself sitting at the table "done in." Several hours of relative immobility passed before she yielded to her husband's urging that she call their family doctor. She was told to come to the office, avoiding the gantlet of the local hospital's emergency department.

Dr. S. saw Mrs. K. expeditiously after she arrived. Brow furrowed, the doctor fired off a series of questions about this experience, all of which elicited a negative response. Brow still furrowed by diagnostic thoughts, some of which she mumbled aloud, Dr. S. announced that she was sending Mrs. K. through the emergency department for a series of tests. There followed a long afternoon as Mrs. K. marched from pillar to post, experiencing more and more pain with every transfer, before arriving more exhausted and in even more intense pain to a resting posture on a litter with Dr. S. by her side.

"There aren't any clues to anything going on in your lungs, spinal cord, nerves, bowel, or heart," the doctor told her. "The X-ray is not abnormal, but I suspect you have suffered a tiny fracture of one of the spine bones in the middle of your back. Since there was no unusual trauma, we call this a fragility fracture from your osteoporosis."

That diagnosis struck fear in Mrs. K.'s heart. "You told me I had osteopenia ten years ago," she said. "I've been on Fosamax ever since, and you told me my bone density had improved. Are you certain I have a spine fracture?"

The answer was yes, but there was nothing reassuring about this diagnosis. The diagnosis is a horror in the minds of all American women, calling forth the images of repeated painful fractures, a stooped and unsightly posture, and withering. Dr. S. tried to reassure Mrs. K. that the fracture should heal well over the next week or two. To tide her over, she offered a prescription for oxycodone, which Mrs. K.'s husband filled on their way home.

Dreadful weeks passed, and then more weeks. Daytime was barely tolerable, but Mrs. K. was a trouper. She managed to dress on her own and usually could stand from the toilet without help from her husband. He helped her slip into the passenger seat so that she could get out of the house. Getting out of the car was a challenge. Her universe was dramatically constrained by mechanical pain, pain induced by any alteration in posture.

Nighttime was worse. Mrs. K. was comfortable recumbent with a couple of pillows, but if she moved, she was jolted awake. The toilette became an enemy, and not just because it was so difficult to sit and stand. She was constipated and was having difficulty initiating urination, symptoms that Dr. S. ascribed to the narcotics and for which various potions and pills were added, with some benefit.

Dr. S. saw Mrs. K. frequently. Empathy, concern, and a wavering of her "you'll be better soon" pronouncements characterized these visits. Fortunately, nothing new was going on. At week ten, Dr. S. suggested a referral for vertebroplasty. This is a procedure where the radiologist identifies the fractured vertebra and injects it with a substance that hardens like cement, solidifying the fracture. Mrs. K. was desperate, so off she went. She suffered through the MRI and was told that indeed it appeared that one particular vertebral body was changed in a fashion that indicated bone damage. That vertebra was subsequently injected, and she began to rapidly improve. Two weeks later, she was capable of her customary activities of daily living, but not quite capable of thinking of herself as any longer in her Golden Years. Mrs. K.'s sense of invincibility was more fragile than her vertebrae.

This vignette is a fearsome specter for all adult women in America and to a lesser extent women elsewhere, and if "health promotion" has its way, it will become increasingly frightening for men as well. And Mrs. K.'s spinal fragility fracture is the least of the specter. How about hip fractures? Almost every pronouncement about osteoporosis that is published in the lay or clinical literature starts with some horrifying estimate of the prevalence of spinal fragility fractures, such as they occur in over half of women over fifty.[1] We are offered and marketed a growing menu of options, largely pharmaceutical options, to hold the horror at bay. How many of us are aware that nearly all of these spinal fragility fractures go unrecognized by the people who have them?[2]

I have long pointed to osteoporosis as one of the best examples of disease mongering by the pharmaceutical industry,[3] and I'm no longer alone in doing so.[4] The thinning of our bones is a risk factor that has been turned into a horrifying disease that must be thwarted, regardless of the cost or the risk. Shouldn't one try to toughen the bones before they collapse? Hence, many well women are offered or seek quantification of their "bone mineral density" (BMD), only to learn that they are not as well as they had thought. So many learn when they're young that they are fragile and will be even more fragile after menopause. I have also long argued that we have no right to medicalize women, or menopause, or aging in this fashion. Medicalization redefines nonmedical problems as diseases or disorders that require medical intervention when there is no reason to assert that such intervention is beneficial. Is gray hair a disease? Medicalization is all too common and all too costly.[5]

Mrs. K. has long been medicalized, and Dr. S. has been swept up in the "standard of care" that all too often is the product of disease mongering, which is so highly orchestrated as to be nefarious. It worked to establish the standard of care for normalizing blood sugar or cholesterol. Let me explain how it works for "dem bones, dem bones . . ."

Osteopenia and Osteoporosis

Bone is a living tissue. That means it is forever growing, but in a regulated fashion, so the cells in the bone remove the old at the same rate that they produce the new. Bone grows in size into our teens. Adult bone continues to grow stronger into our thirties. That doesn't mean we are taller, but that there is more bone and better-mineralized bone per given volume.

Many hormonal mechanisms are invested in bone health. Physical forces and activity contribute to this balance into our fifties, when we head into negative balance, slowly losing bone mineral and the bone itself over the next decades. This negative balance is much more marked in women after menopause than ever in men. But all this is normal aging. It is the graying of our bone. It is still bone health. Our aging bones lose more than their substance, however; they lose resilience and are not as resistant to fracture as they once were. Furthermore, the plateau we reach in our thirties is not the same for all of us. Normally, healthy women arrive at a plateau in their thirties that has less bone and less mineral density than men. Normally, white and Asian women arrive at even less than other women. Therefore, since the bone mineral density goes south after menopause, elderly white women are prone to particularly fragile bones. We've known this for generations. Until 1993 osteoporosis could be diagnosed only when someone had a fragility fracture, particularly a spinal fragility fracture that was apparent on X-ray. The reason for this is illustrated in Figures 6 and 7.

That all changed when X-ray machines were adapted to measure BMD. Here was a metric that spoke to the toughness of a bone and the degree to which it was at risk for fragility fractures. BMD was swept into the risk-factor maelstrom along with all else we've considered. The World Health Organization (WHO) procured pharmaceutical funding to convene a study group that in 1994 produced a document setting forth the stochastic relationship between BMD and the incidence of fragility fractures.[6] Essentially, they took the average BMD for young men and for young women and said if a person is more than 2.5 standard deviations below that average, they have osteoporosis. This is stated as a "T score," and −2.5 defines osteoporosis with or without an extant fragility fracture. Furthermore, if a person is between 1.0 and 2.5 standard deviations below the mean (a T score between −1 and −2.5), they are on their way to osteoporosis because they have a lesser amount of mineralized bone. This condition was called osteopenia.

The development of risk assessment coincided with the introduction of bisphosphonates, first etidronate (Didronel) and then alendronate (Fosamax). These are agents that can cause bone mineral density to increase measurably. Merck & Company wasted no time in inserting Fosamax into common practice, if not common sense. After all, a "low" BMD was a risk and a "very low" BMD a pressing risk for fragility fractures. Shouldn't we treat the BMD with the expectation that doing so will ameliorate the

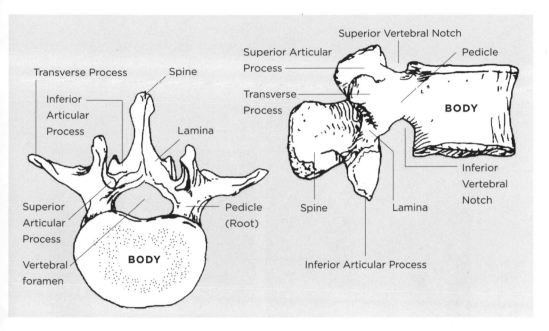

Figure 6. These diagrams offer some of the anatomical detail that underlies Mrs. K.'s fragility fracture. The perspective in the left-hand drawing is looking down the spine from the skull at a vertebra. The spinal canal (vertebral foramen) is obvious, as are the structures that delineate this space. The vertebral bodies and the discs between them are the floor of the canal, the pedicles are the walls, and the posterior elements are the roof.

The diagram on the right correlates with Frame B of Figure 7, the side view. You can see the spine, or spinous process, of the spine protruding back from the posterior elements. You can also see structures in the posterior elements protruding up, toward the head, and down to form joints with the adjacent vertebrae that allow motion and contribute to the stability of the spinal column.

However, the weight-bearing function of the spine largely belongs to the column of vertebral bodies and the discs between them. The vertebral body is bone. The outer rim is dense bone; the center is a filigree of bone. As we age, the depth of the rim tends to shrink. However, more dramatically, the lacework that makes up the filigree in the center becomes composed less and less of bone, with each element itself growing thinner. The vertebral body becomes more fragile, with a tendency to collapse in the center, taking on the shape of the vertebral bodies of many fish; or it may collapse opposite the spinous process, taking on a wedge shape.

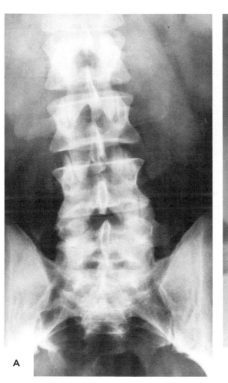

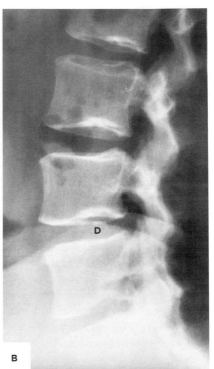

Figure 7. These X-rays are like those that Dr. S. described as normal. X-rays are like photographs, but they use X-rays instead of light to affect the film. The efficiency with which X-rays penetrate through the body depends on the type of tissue they encounter; the denser the tissue, the less they can pass through and the more the image appears white. Well-mineralized, dense bone blocks the X-rays and appears white, whereas air-containing tissues appear black. Shades of gray speak to the varying density of the tissues. Hence, the rim of the vertebral bodies looks white because of its dense bone, in contrast to the gray of the center with its bony filigree. As the vertebral bodies become osteoporotic, the contrast is more striking. That's not only because there is less bone, but also because the bone that's there has less calcium. Calcium is the principal mineral of bone and the principal cause of bony density. "Bone Mineral Density" determinations (BMD) take advantage of the degree to which X-rays can pass through bone; the more readily they pass, the less dense the bone.

In Frame A, the view is as if you were looking through the belly at the spine; Frame B is the view from the side. In Frame A, the vertebral bodies are the rectangular shadows that seem to be floating. The dense elliptical structures in the midline are the spinous processes that protrude from the center of the posterior elements; these are the bumps we can feel with our fingers in the middle of our backs. In Frame B, the vertebral bodies appear squarer and can be seen to be attached by bone to the posterior elements. The space between the vertebral bodies appears empty and black, but it is anything but empty. The vertebral bodies are connected by a complex soft tissue, the disc. (I've placed a *D* in one of the disc "spaces.")

This is the image of a relatively pristine spine. In someone the age of Mrs. K., such a pristine spine would be highly unusual. Rather, there would be changes in the composition of discal tissue: disc spaces would be narrow and degenerative changes commonplace around the vertebral bodies and the posterior elements, including the formation of spurs and the like. Changes in the vertebral body itself are also guaranteed, with a decrease in the density of the rim and central bone. These may be very hard to discern on a routine X-ray, since they may present as little more than an increase in contrast between the whiteness of the rim and the grayness of the center of the vertebral body. That is true if collapse of the center or of the rim is subtle. In such a case, one can use Magnetic Resonance Imaging (MRI) to see if there is a change in the composition of the bone itself.

risk, thereby sparing us fragility fractures? In the United States, universal screening of older women by BMD is recommended. As is true of all the screening modalities we have examined, BMD has not escaped critical thinking unscathed. I'm not sure the same holds for the willingness of physicians to prescribe bisphosphonates, the desire of women to know their BMD, or the compliance of women with prescriptions for bisphosphonates.

HOW WELL DOES BMD PREDICT FRAGILITY FRACTURES?

In the scientific community, it is well known that BMD is only one of many risk factors for fragility fractures. For example, no matter her T score, a fifty-year-old woman has a far lower likelihood of a fragility fracture in the next decade than a seventy-year-old woman with the same T score.[7] That's true even if both women have a T score of −2.5 or less. Furthermore, any who has had a fragility fracture is at greater risk for another, regardless of her or his T score. Advanced age and a prior fragility fracture are harbingers that have been obvious for generations. Of course, the grail of risk-factor epidemiology is to find others at risk, even at low risk with osteopenia, and treat them early. After all, the number of people who are osteopenic is enormous, so effectively treating all of them helps only a small fraction — but a small fraction of a very large population, meaning that many more people are spared than if only the very old with T scores of −2.5 or less are treated.[8] Because of this grail, screening and treating has a life of its own in practice and in the lay press in America.

In academic circles, there is much grumbling over the poor predictive value of a diagnosis of osteopenia. Other aspects of bone physiology are at least as crucial as BMD in determining the strength of bones. Some of these factors are not inherent to bone strength.[9] One such factor is neuromuscular health. Seldom does a normal bone directly feel the force applied to the body. For example, the forces of heel strike during walking or those of bending over and lifting a box are not directly transmitted to the spine; these forces are diffused by coordinated muscular activity from the point of application. Such considerations don't lend themselves readily to screening modalities. The epidemiologists who are committed to improving screening by BMD must content themselves with more traditional measures in the quest for the subset of people with osteopenia who are at particularly high risk for fragility fractures.

The latest innovation by the screening club is FRAX, a Web-based computer model that takes into account multiple easily measured risk factors to enhance the predictive value of the BMD. It was introduced by the World Health Organization Metabolic Bone Disease Group based on an analysis of multiple epidemiological cohort studies.[10] The risk factors that the FRAX model incorporates are age, sex, fracture history, use of oral steroids, presence of rheumatoid arthritis or other specified conditions associated with secondary osteoporosis, smoking status, family history of a hip fracture, early menopause, low BMI, and excessive alcohol consumption. The International Osteoporosis Foundation and the National Osteoporosis Foundation in the United States now recommend treating adults over fifty if their BMD score is osteopenic and they are predicted to have a ten-year probability of hip fracture of 3 percent or higher and of any osteoporotic fracture of 20 percent or higher, based on FRAX. FRAX has infused enthusiasm for, and self-righteousness back into, the osteopenia screening enterprise, even though it performs much better for hip fractures (see below) than other fragility fractures.[11] Furthermore, it is not clear that it offers any more predictive value than much simpler models such as age and BMD alone, or for that matter age and fracture history alone.[12] We know that.

To restate the mantra, one never wants to submit to screening unless the test is accurate, the disease is important, and we can do something about it. Screening by BMD for the risk of fragility fractures fails on all scores. It is basically an expensive way to ask a thin white or Asian woman her age. It works best when one has already had a fragility fracture, but that's a tautology. It also works when one has secondary osteoporosis, secondary to any of a number of readily diagnosed disease and drug toxicities—but that's obvious, too. Does the "disease," osteopenia, carry sufficient risk that the diagnosis should trigger intervention? The most common fragility fractures are at the spine and cannot be distinguished from all the other episodes of axial pain that plague all of us frequently and the elderly more frequently. Most fragility fractures are a disease without a specific illness; they are part of normal aging. Furthermore, they are not the principal reason for the loss of height and the stooped posture Mrs. K. dreads. Height loss is more a function of disc degeneration and gait disorders than compression of vertebral bodies.

And the stooped posture, so-called dowager's hump, is often not a result of compression fractures. The dorsal spine (the spine in the back of the chest) is normally convex, so we are all a bit hunched. The tendency of the dorsal spine to be convex is termed kyphosis. Some of us are more hunched over than others throughout adult life, which elicits the "stand up straight" admonition more than the abnormal label. And some of us become more and more hunched through adult life, so that more than 20 percent of elderly people qualify for a label—hyperkyphosis—that denotes abnormality.[13] Occasionally, this is so extreme that lung function is compromised. However, only about a third of the elderly with hyperkyphosis have underlying fragility fractures. We have no good understanding as to why/how hyperkyphosis develops. Degenerative changes in the discs contribute. There may be a neuromuscular contribution that involves an imbalance over time between muscles that pull us forward and those that hold us back. There is a form that I observed while teaching in Japan, a common condition where the kyphosis reverses with recumbency as if this is a weakness of the muscles that hold one erect. But hyperkyphosis generally does not reverse with recumbency; it is a rigid deformity for which the treatment of osteoporosis offers little hope.

Could it be that we're doing little more than medicalizing aging?

WHY DID MRS. K.'S FRAGILITY FRACTURE HURT?

Wait a minute, you say. There is nothing "normal" about Mrs. K.'s nightmarish experience. Maybe it's the extreme, but it's the nightmare of "osteoporosis" come true, with the promise of more grief to come. She and Dr. S. managed ten weeks of forbearance before seeking cure from vertebroplasty. There's a lesson in this that will probably come as a surprise.

Vertebroplasty was introduced over a decade ago. It seemed like a good idea, and all the widgets were in place. Interventional radiologists are trained to stick needles in lots of secret places in the body; hitting a vertebral body is elementary. The "cement" is the same compound long used for gluing artificial hips and knees in place and therefore is known to be nontoxic. Intrepid interventional radiologists could not contain themselves. Neither Institutional Review Boards nor the FDA need sanction such an activity since all they were doing is common practice adapted to a different bone. Before long, Medicare was purchasing some 40,000 vertebroplasties every year simply because their advisory panels bowed to the cogent arguing of the interventional radiology community. After all, these interventionalists were able to point to more than one dramatic response to the procedure akin to Mrs. K.'s.

Then, in the summer of 2009, two randomized sham-controlled trials of vertebroplasty were published in the *New England Journal of Medicine*. Both trials were federally supported, not industry supported. In both, patients had persistent symptoms similar to Mrs. K.'s. In both, local an-

TABLE 4

Principal Results of the Australian Randomized Sham-Controlled Trial of Vertebroplasty (All Figures Percentages)

Perceived Pain	ONE WEEK		ONE MONTH	
	Vertebroplasty	Sham	Vertebroplasty	Sham
Better	16	35	34	24
No change	70	62	60	53
Worse	14	3	6	24

Mrs. K. was one of about a third of patients who are helped by undergoing a "procedure" rather than from vertebroplasty.

Source: R. Buchbinder, R. H. Osborne, P. R. Ebeling, et al., A randomized trial of vertebroplasty for painful osteoporotic vertebral fractures, *New England Journal of Medicine* 2009; 361: 557–68.

esthesia was applied with a needle inserted near the fractured vertebral body, but the vertebral body was entered and the cement injected in only half the patients. The patients and the doctors who followed their progress were not apprised of which treatment was performed. Vertebroplasty did not result in any significant advantage in pain or function over the sham procedure at any point over the next six months.[14] That means that Mrs. K. was as likely to come away from the sham procedure smiling as from the vertebroplasty (Table 4).

Mrs. K. was one of about a third of patients who are better having a "procedure." How do we get our minds around such a "placebo effect"? I can assure you that if Dr. S. had said, "I want to send you over to my friendly interventional radiologist for a sham procedure," the likelihood that Mrs. K. would even go, let alone have a 35 percent chance of improvement, is nil. I can also assure you that Mrs. K. is not "nuts," or feigning, or malingering, or driven by secondary gains such as manipulating Mr. K. And I can assure you that the local anesthetic did not account for more than hours of benefit, if any. The lesson of Mrs. K.'s vertebroplasty relates to the difference between pain and suffering. Pain is hardwired and aversive, sometimes unspeakably beyond description. Suffering is the intellectualization of the experience of pain. Pain that is comprehensible, explicable, and predictably self-limited engenders less suffering—otherwise no woman would have a second child. That's why dental pain, fractures, and the like are easier to cope with than low back pain. Such pain is responsive to opiates (narcotics), but often none are deemed necessary since cure or healing is anticipated and coping seems reasonable. But when the pain engenders uncertainty and triggers negative preconceptions, it has suffering as its handmaiden. It is suffering that can be rethought, that is susceptible to a "placebo effect." It is suffering that is enhanced when uncertainty as to prognosis escalates and hope erodes. Mrs. K. paid quite a price for the preconceptions that result from disease mongering, and Dr. S. helped her little with the prescription of oxycodone, which reinforced fears as to the seriousness of the prognosis and added the obligate adverse effects of opiates in elderly people. Nonopiate analgesics, water exercises, support of family members, and smiles from physicians usually suffice to tide people through the healing of a symptomatic vertebral compression fracture once everyone is convinced that this, too, shall pass.

What are we to do about vertebroplasty? Another, smaller trial came up with the same result but with a hint that injecting the cement had some sort of acute, fleeting palliative effect.[15] But that hardly justifies this expensive procedure, which has well-described potential for serious side effects. The response of the vertebroplasty-performing interventional radiology community to these trials was hardly gentle, finding fault with the design of the trials, particularly their selection criteria.[16] It's reminiscent of the interventional cardiology community's response to the stenting trials.

I tend to be charitable regarding the reflex to "protest too much." In chapter 3, I discussed the folly of peer review. Franklin Miller and David Kallmes argue that these interventionalists are so convinced they are doing well by the patient that their conviction is the agent of the placebo effect rather than their procedure.[17] Nonetheless, their conviction is as unshakable as that of the interventional cardiologists who place stents, and their collective voices make it difficult to halt their practice despite the fact that it flies in the face of best evidence. One leading spine surgeon chimed in with the "careful patient selection is paramount"[18] argument, while another stopped short of calling for a halt of reimbursement, preferring to "empower" the patient to decline the procedure.[19] The response of a leading health-services researcher is to take advantage of the seldom-used ability of the Medicare administration to reimburse only if patients are entered into a registry so that benefits can be discerned going forward.[20] My approach is to cease reimbursing until benefit is demonstrated and to inform the public at large as to the rationale I've just set before the reader. Maybe we will see a shift in our culture, so that technology will not be valued for technology's sake and the FDA will be empowered to see that is so.

DO BISPHOSPHONATES DO ANY GOOD?

Every licensed bisphosphonate increases BMD, even in postmenopausal women for whom the loss of BMD is a fact of life. There are a lot of postmenopausal women, and many of them are at risk for fragility fractures, mainly vertebral fragility fractures. The pharmaceutical industry was quick to recognize both facts, quick to seek drugs that can serve this enormous population, quicker to market such, and slower to study whether the women are better off for the activity. But decades have gone by, and we are inundated with data from randomized controlled trials. When the American College of Physicians produced its treatment guidelines to prevent fragility fractures in 2008,[21] the committee had well over 400 randomized controlled trials to rely on. Many of these trials were attempts to show that the agents actually prevented vertebral fragility fractures rather than simply raise BMD. Many were attempting to demonstrate protection from nonvertebral fractures, which is a far more demanding exercise as these are far less common. Many were "seed trials" designed mainly to familiarize large numbers of clinicians and their patients with a particular agent. Some were attempts to show that my bisphosphonate is better than yours. In fact, much of the "advances" are in terms of how often the pills have to be taken, an issue in convenience and for compliance.

Every licensed bisphosphonate has now been shown to decrease the incidence of vertebral fragility fractures. Before you exclaim "Wow," realize that this is a radiological result. A vertebral fragility fracture is usually defined as a 20 percent decrease in the height of a vertebra, which is usually about 2 millimeters and not so easy to discern on these X-rays (Figure 7). Rarely do the investigators have the temerity to suggest that they can eke out of the data any decrease in the incidence of back pain. So, every licensed bisphosphonate can treat X-ray images. As I mentioned earlier, these fractures are not the principal reason we lose height or become stooped as we age.

The newest bisphosphonate on the block is zoledronic acid (Zometa). It's the one you literally hear about all the time, thanks to Novartis's marketing team. Table 5 presents the principal results of the HORIZON Pivotal Fracture Trial.[22] This was a three-year, double-blind, placebo-controlled multicenter international trial sponsored by Novartis. Almost 4,000 women were recruited; their average age was seventy-three and

TABLE 5
Principal Results of the HORIZON Trial of Zoledronic Acid

Outcome	Zoledronic Acid (%)	Placebo (%)	Relative Risk Reduction (%)	Number Needed to Treat to Help One Person
Vertebral fracture	3.3	11	70	14
Hip fracture	1.4	2.5	41	98
Nonvertebral fracture	8.0	11	25	38
Any clinical fracture	8.4	14	33	24
Stroke	2.3	2.3	1.4	—
			Relative Risk Increase (%)	Number Needed to Treat to Harm One Person
Any adverse event	95.5	93.9	1.7	62
Serious atrial fibrillation	1.3	0.5	149	129

almost all had a T score of less than −2.5 at the hip. Furthermore, two-thirds already had at least one vertebral fragility fracture when the trial started. So this was a trial of treating elderly women who already had osteoporosis by WHO criteria, and most had it by clinical criteria. This is a trial of secondary prevention. Remember, older women with a prior fragility fracture are at the highest risk for another fragility fracture. You should not assume that the results would be the same for women with osteopenia or even for women with a T score less than −2.5 who have yet to fracture.

This very high-risk group had an 11 percent incidence of morphometric (determined by measuring the height of the vertebral body on X-rays), radiographic (usually asymptomatic) vertebral fragility fractures, which dropped by 8 percent if they were on zoledronic acid. That is not a trivial result statistically, but one needs to keep the perspective that almost none of these women knew the X-ray image of their spine had changed. It's the rest of the table that is cause for debate, if not concern.

Yes, there was a reduction in the incidence of hip fractures, and hip fractures are always of grave concern (see below). It is usually marketed as a 41 percent reduction in hip fractures, but you know better; that's the relative reduction. The actual reduction is 1 percent, meaning we have to give this agent to 100 women for three years to stand a chance of sparing one of them a hip fracture. Before any elderly woman with osteoporosis agrees to this treatment, they should understand that this is the degree to which they might be advantaged. The results in Table 5 were generated in the HORIZON trial, but the results of all the many trials for the alternative bisphosphonates are similar;[23] many can't even generate this puny benefit in terms of hip fractures.

DO BISPHOSPHONATES DO ANY HARM?

Bone health requires the orchestrated turnover of bone. There are cells dedicated to degrading bone — the osteoclasts — and cells dedicated to restoring it — the osteoblasts. The bisphosphonates largely interfere with the function of the osteoclasts, thereby pushing the balance toward formation of bone. One of the first bisphosphonates on the market was etidronate (Didronel). We soon learned that it was a double-edged sword in that, if used too long, it also interfered with the quality of new bone and led to fragility fractures. Another early bisphosphonate was introduced to stop cancer-cell metastases from growing in bone; that didn't last long because leukemia was a complication. Ever since, we have been wary of these agents. That's why the recent report of atypical fractures of the femur (the thigh bone) raised eyebrows[24] and caused the radiologists involved in so many of the trials to return to the X-rays looking for these atypical fractures. They found no increase,[25] which should be interpreted as indicating they are quite rare. Since the decrease in the incidence of hip fractures is a tenuous clinical benefit of bisphosphonate treatment, one would hardly consider any important increase in the incidence of femoral fractures a rational trade-off. While there is debate about whether femoral fractures can be ascribed to bisphosphonates, none remains about osteonecrosis of the jaw.[26] This is a rare but horrific complication that is seen only with bisphosphonates; the bone of the jaw dies requiring extensive reconstructive surgery. The statin Baycol was removed from the market because it, too, caused a rare but horrific complication (muscle necrosis) that rendered seeking its putative benefit unacceptably risky.

These are the nightmares that should plague any physician who prescribed bisphosphonates without being able to generate a cogent rationale. There are other adverse effects that are more common. One is the last column in Table 5: serious atrial fibrillation. This is a disturbance that causes the rhythm of the heart to become rapid and chaotic, often causing the patient considerable distress and requiring intervention. It is about as likely an untoward outcome in this elderly population as the secondary prevention of hip fractures is a positive outcome from zoledronic acid treatments. It occurs with other bisphosphonates, including alendronate.[27] Speaking of alendronate, it's toxic to the lining of the esophagus, so women have to go to lengths to swallow it more safely.

By the way, men do not escape the radar of all this disease mongering. Because the rate of loss of BMD with aging differs by gender, far fewer men arrive at anyone's definition of osteopenia, let alone osteoporosis. But some do. Furthermore, once a man has a fragility fracture, the risk of a subsequent fracture is similar to that of women.[28] The American College of Physicians' guidelines for screening men are similar to its guidelines for women.[29] The wrinkle with men is that low-trauma fractures are more likely to be rib fractures.[30] Of course, all the caveats regarding treatment pertain to men.

ALTERNATIVES TO BISPHOSPHONATES

Long before there were the bisphosphonates, there was hormone replacement therapy (HRT). I discuss HRT in great detail in *Worried Sick* and will not reiterate the arguments here since so little has changed and so much is overblown. All I will say is that if you didn't decide to pop these pills well before age sixty-five, there's little reason to do so after.[31] There is a steady stream of new Specific Estrogen Receptor Modulators (SERMS) that are designed to target bone health. These have their own side effects and are no more effective than the bisphosphonates. As for older men, testosterone supplementation will do nothing discernible to prevent decline in cognition or BMD and may be harmful.[32] Supplementation with the adrenal sex hormone DHEA has physiologic effects in the direction of the "fountain-of-youth," but they are trivial for elderly men and for women.[33]

A great deal of science and money has been invested in figuring out how to get parathyroid hormone to help with osteoporosis. It is a very powerful hormone that regulates bone turnover, causing far too much bone destruction if overproduced. There are forms of parathyroid hormone and doses that have just the other effect.[34] Two of these are now clinically available and quite expensive. They are no more effective than we've seen for the bisphosphonates, however. Furthermore, no one has been able to show that combining these various classes of drugs designed to increase BMD leads to an additive effect. Rather, if one has a fragility fracture while being treated with a drug of one class, it is common practice to switch to a drug of another.

This brings us to the latest fountain-of-youth hormone: vitamin D. Yes, vitamin D is a hormone. Sunlight causes its precursor to be made from substances in the skin. The precursor travels to the liver, where it is partially activated, and on to the kidney to be fully activated. The principal target for activated vitamin D is the gut. Without activated vitamin D, we absorb calcium very poorly. And blood/tissue *calcium* is the name of the game. Normal body chemistry is very dependent on the amount of calcium bathing our cells. A great deal of body metabolism is invested in keeping our calcium level rock stable. There are two sources of calcium for this purpose: bone and food. Mobilizing calcium from bone is an effect of parathyroid hormone; absorbing calcium from food is the effect of activated vitamin D. These two hormones play off one another. If the blood calcium is tending to fall, the parathyroid gland is stimulated to produce more parathyroid hormone, which increases resorption of bone and also increases the efficiency of the activation of vitamin D by the kidney. If the calcium is tending to rise, the opposite happens. That's why it's so difficult to raise body calcium, let alone BMD, by ingesting calcium salts; unless there's too much activated vitamin D, you're treating the toilette bowl. None of the over-the-counter vitamin D preparations are the activated form, which is why it takes a great deal over the recommended dietary requirements to see an effect of dietary supplementation; the vitamin is absorbed but not activated if blood calcium is adequate. Overdosing can overwhelm this elegant servomechanism. But most vitamin D and calcium supplementation is a waste of money.

That's actually true for the FDA's required supplementation of dairy products. Most of us do not need to ingest any vitamin D. After all, if you're fair skinned, you will make your daily requirements yourself with less than an hour of exposing your arms and face to sunlight a few times a week. But not everyone is fair skinned, and not everyone gets that much sun exposure. Between limited sunlight, air pollution, and lifestyle, the British were faced with an epidemic of the kind of bone disease that results from too little vitamin D and therefore too little absorption of dietary calcium. The special bone disease that results from vitamin D deficiency is not osteoporosis (too little bone) but osteomalacia—rickets in childhood—where there is plenty of bone but it is poorly mineralized and fragile on that basis. The solution was to supplement vitamin D in commercially prepared dairy products. All resource-advantaged countries supplement their commercial dairy products with enough vitamin

D to avoid dietary deficiency but not too much to risk overwhelming the servomechanism and causing too high a calcium level.

So who needs vitamin D supplementation beyond this public-health solution? No one does if their diet is replete with dairy products or if they have sufficient sun exposure. There are groups of people who may have neither—the institutionalized elderly for one. How about most of us? How about most of us over age sixty-five? Have we been too complacent about requirements? And what is there to lose? These nagging questions have inserted themselves into the "health promotion" construct so that vitamin D and calcium have long had a prominent place on every grocer's health-foods shelf to promote bone health and avoid fragility fractures. These nagging questions have also occupied a number of investigators for a number of years. Heike Bischoff-Ferrari and colleagues were able to collect twelve randomized controlled trials,[35] all double-blind (neither the person handing out the pills nor the person swallowing the pills knew if the pill was vitamin D or a placebo). They concluded: "Nonvertebral fracture prevention with vitamin D is dose dependent, and a higher dose should reduce fractures by at least 20 percent for individuals aged 65 years or older." By now, every reader knows to be leery of a relative risk reduction assertion without knowing the absolute risk reduction (Table 6).

I am not a fan of what we can learn from meta-analyses for reasons that this table exemplifies. First, realize that no one does a meta-analysis unless there is a sizeable literature on a particular topic dripping small, and often conflicting, results. The intent of the meta-analysis is somehow to merge all of these experiences to produce a greater truth. In doing a meta-analysis, the investigators cull from the literature every randomized controlled trial they can find and discard those that they deem too methodologically unsound to be informative. This is the one of several subjective aspects to the exercise; criteria are crafted to settle differences when one investigator's unsound trial is another's joy to behold. They next examine the acceptable trials and weight them as to quality, so that the acceptable trial that is deemed the most methodologically sound will carry the greatest weight. Again, this is a subjective exercise to decide whether a trial that had lots of subjects drop out but is otherwise perfect is more valuable than a trial that had a flaw in randomization but is otherwise perfect. You get the idea: the meekest investigator does not have the last say. Then the investigators attempt to merge the data, which requires multiple assumptions. For me, the results of any meta-analysis are never as interesting as the fact that someone thought a meta-analysis was nec-

TABLE 6

Meta-Analysis of Trials of Vitamin D Supplementation to Prevent Fragility Fractures in Well People over Age Sixty-Five

VITAMIN D DOSE 340–380 IU/DAY
DURATION OF OBSERVATION 24–62 MONTHS

Number of Subjects	Rate of Nonvertebral Fractures (D v. Placebo)		Rate of Hip Fractures (D v. Placebo)		Relative Risk Reduction	Number Needed to Treat to Spare One an Event
9,014	12%	12%			2%	Not significant
9,014			4.5%	4.1%	9%	Not significant

VITAMIN D DOSE 482–770 IU/DAY
DURATION OF OBSERVATION 12–84 MONTHS

Number of Subjects	Rate of Nonvertebral Fractures (D v. Placebo)		Rate of Hip Fractures (D v. Placebo)		Relative Risk Reduction	Number Needed to Treat to Spare One an Event
33,265	4.4%	5.5%			20%	93
31,872			2.7%	3.2%	18%	168

essary; I find this symbolic of "much ado about exceedingly little." That is how I interpret the results in Table 6, and I fault the investigators for the hubris to mislead the readership with a conclusion of a "20 percent reduction" in events. I'm not surprised that another analysis of these and other vitamin D fracture trials could not eke out any advantage to vitamin D alone but massaged an absolute reduction over three years of less than 1 percent if the vitamin D was combined with calcium.[36] Much ado about nothing.

But in our culture, the notion that a supplement has nothing to do with health dies slowly, if ever. I've offered an overview of the critical role vitamin D plays in calcium homeostasis. Other minor roles have emerged from the study of human biology, but many effects have emerged from studying various biologic systems in test tubes. These latter observations have fostered myriad hypotheses for therapeutic roles of vitamin D other than to toughen bones. One is to diminish the consequences of falls in the elderly. Multiple trials have been undertaken, with inconsistent small effects found; the conclusion from two meta-analyses[37] is that there may be a small protective effect to high doses of vitamin D, particularly high doses of an active vitamin D metabolite. Then Kerrie Sanders and her colleagues published the results of a randomized controlled trial of administered high doses of an active D metabolite each winter to over 2,000 community-dwelling women over age seventy.[38] The women who received the supplement fell a little bit more frequently. Caveat emptor.

The claims for potential benefits of vitamin D supplementation seem boundless: cardiovascular disease, diabetes, rheumatic diseases, cancer, and on and on. Furthermore, the common methodologies for measuring vitamin D are scaled so that more and more "deficiencies" are diagnosed and more and more people are swallowing supplemental vitamin D. It's reminiscent of the antioxidant zeal a decade ago. That came to an end when the science matured so that the data that demonstrated a degree of harm overwhelmed the data that suggested a degree of benefit.[39] I suspect the zeal for vitamin D supplementation will suffer a similar fate. Already, a committee of experts convened by the Institute of Medicine has concluded that there is no need for additional D or calcium supplementation and pursuing such may prove harmful.[40]

HIP FRACTURES

Mrs. K. aside, vertebral fragility fractures are not themselves a pressing public-health issue in comparison to fragility fractures in general and hip fractures in particular. Fragility fractures mark a segment of the aging population who are at significantly increased risk of death—for all-cause mortality—compared to others in their birth cohorts who have not suffered any fragility fracture.[41] This association is most marked for low-trauma hip fractures. Older adults have a five- to eightfold increased risk of dying during the first three months after the fracture. Excess annual mortality persists afterward, more so for men.[42] Realize that orthopedic surgery is a match for these hip fractures; the commonest procedure, pinning the fracture, is relatively straightforward and not that traumatic, even for the frail. It is nowhere near the trauma of abdominal surgery or cardiac surgery. Yet despite rapidly "fixing" the fracture and rehabilitating the patient, the mortality hazard persists. Clearly, low-trauma hip fractures are a manifestation of impending or current debility. The good news is that the age-standardized rates of low-trauma hip fractures have steadily declined. That means they are occurring at older ages, when the mortal hazard that can be ascribed to the fracture is subsumed by all-cause mortality.[43] Debility is moving toward the end of our natural life span.

Nonetheless, nonvertebral, low-trauma fractures are major, miserable events at any age, and vertebral fragility fractures can be comparably evil—as Mrs. K. discovered. In Mrs. K.'s case, the "low-trauma" was unavoidable (just sitting up in bed). But hip, wrist, and shoulder fractures usually result from slips and falls. The older we are, the less likely we are to simply get up, brush ourselves off, and start all over again—sometimes because of decrepitude and sometimes because of a fractured bone. Given the dismal track record of all the pharmaceutical efforts at strengthening bones, another approach has been vying for center stage: preventing falls.[44] Some of the interventions have obvious face value, such as living space that is barrier free, devoid of obstacles, devoid of slippery surfaces, and replete with handrails. Some are obvious on reflection, such as wearing multifocal glasses on unfamiliar surfaces.[45]

Some will seem obvious once they are pointed out—namely, drugs, and more particularly, drugs that have sedative and hypnotic effects or side effects, such as antidepressants.[46] The most hazardous pharmaceuticals with respect to falling are opiates.[47] This fact, coupled with the observation that elderly persons with chronic musculoskeletal pain are at high risk of falling independent of their medications,[48] is a cogent argument against the prescription of narcotics in this age group. I take strong exception with the recommendations of the American Geriatrics Society in this regard.[49] I agree that modest dosing with acetaminophen is the regimen of choice for musculoskeletal pain management in older people. It has a very favorable benefit/risk ratio, even in the setting of mild kidney disease. I also agree that there is little more to be gained from any nonsteroidal anti-inflammatory drug except the potential for causing any hidden ulcer to bleed. I do not agree that "frequent or continuous pain on a daily basis" is an indication for opiates in the setting of the regional musculoskeletal disorders we are discussing. The panel that composed the American Geriatrics Society guidelines admits that their recommendation is "weak" and based on "low quality" evidence. I'd argue that the evidence for harm overwhelms their weak recommendation. I'd also argue that palliation beyond acetaminophen requires supportive care directed toward enhanced coping and diminished suffering.

Much effort has been expended in learning how to render older persons less susceptible to falling by improving gait and balance through targeted exercise regimens. These can improve physical function and enhance quality of life.[50] But it is not clear that any single intervention can decrease the likelihood of low-trauma fractures. That reflects the enormous clinical variability in the population at risk. Even trials that undertake multifactorial assessments and tailor interventions — with or without external hip protectors — are limited in effectiveness.[51] The most encouraging approach is a study by Mary Tinetti and her colleagues at Yale.[52] In one region of Connecticut, they went to lengths to inform the clinicians and the staff involved in home-care programs and senior centers of the known hazards for falling. They urged these people to assess their patients and to be proactive as seemed appropriate for each person at risk. There was a meaningful reduction in the rates of serious fall-related injuries in the region compared to the rest of the state.

We will learn that the solution for more than the fragility fractures that plague elderly persons can be found in an informed and caring community. As for fragility fractures, it is not clear that screening for osteopenia or even subclinical osteoporosis is as useful. The U.S. Preventive Services Task Force, in a 2010 update, concluded: "Although methods to identify risk for osteoporotic fractures are available and medications to reduce fractures are effective, no trials directly evaluate screening effectiveness, harms and intervals."[53] I see no reason for any well woman to submit to screening for BMD at any age.

It was the best of times, and then the worst, for Mr. K., too.

Mr. K., at seventy-five, was also enjoying his Golden Years. He vigorously participated in the life of his family and his community and had many friends. He played golf occasionally but bocce ball frequently and skillfully. As long as he could remember, he had the occasional back pain or neck pain, rarely knee pain. Some episodes were more severe, causing him to alter his lifestyle, but not for long—certainly not long enough so that he could recall the details. About a year ago, he had a typical recurrence of low back pain. He was comfortable while recumbent, but bending and twisting motions were difficult. Warm showers and an occasional acetaminophen allowed him to get on with life and do most things except play bocce ball. He expected this to pass quickly and be forgotten along with the other episodes.

This didn't pass quickly. It didn't pass at all. In fact, many of the physical things Mr. K. had to do were becoming challenging. But he didn't let on; that was not his style. Besides, Mrs. K. was now suffering from her fragility fracture. He sucked it up and managed somehow to be her primary care-

giver despite his own discomfort. Then Mrs. K. had her hallelujah response to vertebroplasty and rapidly returned to full and independent living. That's when Mr. K. began to realize how much difficulty he was coping with. It was peculiar—different from anything he had experienced before. He was most comfortable sitting still. He could lie down, but he needed to prop himself up to get to sleep. That had not happened before. But walking was his nemesis. He couldn't get very far before he experienced pain in his buttocks and down the back of his thighs, but not as far as his knees. All he could do when this started was find a chair and sit in it. Mrs. K. remarked that he was walking stooped over like an old man. Mr. K. had prided himself in his bearing. This was more than embarrassing; it was an assault on his personal stature and not simply his physical stature.

He didn't notice much else wrong. He was accustomed to urinating at bedtime, immediately on arising, and usually once in the middle of the night. That didn't change. He had little interest in sex and didn't seem to get a morning erection as often. He didn't leap to any concern in that regard. He and Mrs. K. had been abstinent since the onset of her back pain. Prior to that, they had enjoyed much intimacy and frequently enjoyed intercourse. For now, she was busy recovering from, and he coping with, musculoskeletal challenges. Aside from his difficulty walking and the change in posture, he didn't notice much else awry. His weight was stable and his appetite good. It was all about that damnable low back pain.

Dr. S. knew Mr. K. pretty well. She liked him and he her. They were effective together in seeing Mrs. K. through her illness. Besides, he had felt compelled to see Dr. S. annually, even though he felt well and she never found a reason to shake his confidence. He was not one to complain. His present illness caused Dr. S. to furrow her brow yet again. She could elicit nothing additional to add to his narrative of illness. She examined him thoroughly, as she had last year, and found nothing amiss, with the exception of his posture and gait disorder. She mentioned that his pulses were quite full everywhere she knew to feel them and that his neurological examination was entirely reassuring.

Dr. S. pronounced: "I think this is spinal stenosis." She said very little else can present this way. One possibility was a fragility fracture of his pelvis, but that was rare, particularly in men. Another possibility was blockage of some of the branches of the aorta deep in his belly, but that would be highly unusual in someone who had normal pulsations elsewhere. Tumors were unlikely to present this way. "Yup, this is spinal stenosis," she declared. But . . . she wanted a few screening blood and urine tests just to be sure she wasn't

missing something. And she wanted to X-ray his lumbar spine and pelvis—
just ordinary X-rays.

Mr. K. returned the next day to review the results with Dr. S. The blood
and urine tests were normal. She spotted nothing unusual on the X-rays.
There were lots of degenerative changes, lots of spurs and evidence of col-
lapsed discs, but nothing that looked like a tumor was destroying the bone,
which seemed quite well mineralized. They talked.

In 2009 UNC Press published my book *Stabbed in the Back: Confront-ing Back Pain in an Overtreated Society.* It is a comprehensive discussion of the personal, clinical, social, and policy ramifications of regional low back pain. "Regional low back pain" is the backache that afflicts working-age adults who are otherwise well and who have suffered no violent pre-cipitant. A great deal of the monograph is relevant to adults older than typical "working age"—perhaps all except for the discussions relating to work incapacity and its indemnification. None of that is reiterated here. However, *Stabbed in the Back* was not designed to discuss issues that are almost exclusively pertinent to well people after working age. For ex-ample, osteoporosis is not mentioned. Neither is "spinal stenosis." Spinal stenosis has emerged from diagnostic obscurity to be a worry for all aging people without good reason, and to occupy a very contentious perch in the health-care debate with good reason. Does Mr. K. have spinal steno-sis, and what should be done about it?

Spinal Stenosis

Low back pain is ubiquitous. Every culture throughout recorded history has fashioned some line of reasoning regarding its causes, upon which systems of therapy are based. The enormous number of theories and the inventiveness of the therapies is testimony to both the variations of the painful experiences and the inventiveness of thought leaders in each cul-ture. Back pain in elders in the twentieth century West was a low-hanging fruit for this exercise. Depending on how you ask the question, nearly a quarter of people over age seventy have "back symptoms on most days."[54]

It fell to Henk Verbiest to fish the syndrome of spinal stenosis from this sea of morbidity. Verbiest was a highly respected professor of neurosur-gery at Utrecht who, after World War II, was interested in the neurologi-cal disorders that affected children with congenital anomalies that caused narrowing of the spinal canal. Some of the symptoms ascribed to these lesions were reminiscent of the syndrome of "intermittent claudication." Intermittent claudication is a consequence of the buildup of atherosclerotic plaques in the large arteries leading into the legs, so that with exercise, the blood supply is insufficient and the muscles cramp painfully, particularly the calf muscles, causing one to cease walking. It is similar to angina from coronary artery disease. However, the claudication that Verbiest associated with congenital narrowing (or stenosis) of the spinal canal occurred with normal blood vessels and tended to affect the muscles of the buttocks and back of the thighs rather than the calves.

It didn't take long for Verbiest to hear claudicant symptoms in older patients with congenital spinal canal stenosis. Hearing this narrative in the elderly followed. Mr. K. had these classic symptoms, which Verbiest referred to as false claudication (pseudoclaudication) or neurogenic claudication because he inferred that the symptoms were from the spinal cord itself. However, ascribing these symptoms to canal stenosis was problematic in the elderly. Many older spines have lots of degenerative changes that tend to narrow the canal. Verbiest understood early on that canal stenosis and neurogenic claudication could be coincidental, but he was convinced there were nuances that permitted the diagnosis of "spinal stenosis," a specific condition for which surgically widening the canal was a good idea.[55] That was in the mid-1970s.

Between 1979 and 1992, the rate of surgery for spinal stenosis increased eightfold to become the most frequent indication for spine surgery in Medicare recipients. When the clinical experience at major centers was analyzed in 2000, not surprisingly, those patients with the mildest symptoms and the greatest functional capacity had the best outcomes. After all, these are the patients that are likely to do best when treated conservatively and for whom a placebo effect would be predicted if they had been in sham surgical trials such as the vertebroplasty trials discussed before.[56] But there have been no sham surgical trials to date. The most recent attempt at a randomized controlled multicenter trial is plagued by crossovers and dropouts—that is, patients that opted for surgery after assignment to conservative care and patients assigned to surgery who thought better of it.[57] And there is no uniform and accepted definition of neurogenic claudication due to lumbar spinal stenosis.[58] All sorts of patients are operated on or not depending on all sorts of preconceived notions on the part of surgeons and patients. And if the procedure didn't help, the common wisdom suggested that the surgical approach was no match for the magnitude of narrowing.

In the past decade, it has become open season on the elderly back under the banner of "spinal stenosis." Not only that, the inventiveness of the surgical community has been unleashed. More and more of the putatively offending spine was sacrificed to open up the canal, so much that the spine was no longer stable. To compensate for this, surgeons developed new approaches and began to employ more and more hardware to fuse the spine after they'd made it so unstable. Maybe the surgeons strut away after these complex fusion procedures, but their patients are often faced with major complications, including increased thirty-day mortality, and Medicare is faced with burgeoning expenditures.[59] I am not alone in calling for a major change in our thinking about the management of regional back pain in the elderly, with or without pseudoclaudication.[60] A recent systematic review of the literature demonstrates a highly unfavorable risk/benefit ratio.[61] The best you can offer a patient such as Mr. K. is short-term improvement at the price of a challenging recovery and with considerable risks of harm. Medicare should stop underwriting this surgical enterprise until there is an unequivocal demonstration of benefit to some subset in a randomized, sham-controlled trial.

That is not to say that nonsurgical treatments aimed at the spine are an appealing option. The scientific literature on such treatments in older adults is sparse, but the precedents at younger ages are not encouraging. Mr. K. offers the narrative we label "spinal stenosis," a narrative that can call forth a wealth of untested nonsurgical remedies. Before taking any of the bait, Mr. K. should take advantage of Dr. S.'s clinical judgment. Her general impression from the clinical literature is that for many, perhaps a third of the people with his symptoms, the syndrome of spinal stenosis is a mild and self-limited illness. Since that's true for all other regional disorders of the spine despite fixed anatomical abnormalities, including painful fragility fractures, why not hope for such for Mr. K.? Perhaps another third are faced with persistence, and the last third with symptoms that progress in intensity. Dr. S. is also very aware of the interplay between depressive symptoms and back pain. Remember, back pain is a ubiquitous experience and likely to be frequent and more persistent in older people. Elderly people who are depressed are more likely to report back pain and more likely to find that their back pain is disabling.[62] The first line of therapy is directed at maintaining Mr. K.'s sense of humor. As was true for painful fragility fractures, antidepressant and analgesic pharmaceuticals have little to offer, except for adverse effects. Even various activities organized specifically for elderly patients with back pain have little to offer.[63]

Mr. K. needs information as to the illness, particularly its natural history and its limited potential for the unexpected. Mr. K. needs encouragement to get on with his life as best as he can.[64] Bocce ball should be possible since it calls for a stooped posture. Water aerobics likewise can help him maintain his exercise capacity without exacerbating symptoms and, most important, while keeping him integrated into his larger community. And nearly all patients with the syndrome of spinal stenosis can walk unimpaired if leaning over something like a shopping cart or a walker. The latter is stigmatizing, but that mindset needs to be suppressed in favor of mobility. Mobility and community are far more effective at keeping depression at bay than any pharmaceutical.

A Pain in the Neck

A great deal is known about neck pain, but much pertains to working-age adults and not elderly people. We know it is common in the elderly, though not quite as common as low back pain. Then again, musculoskeletal pain somewhere is very common in the elderly, particularly in older women. If you follow a cohort of elderly community-dwelling people closely for a year, over 80 percent will report joint pain somewhere. In fact, pain in more than one location is common, and even widespread pain can afflict as many as 15 percent of women and 5 percent of men. Most of these symptoms will wax and wane over the course of the year. The more that mobility is preserved, the more likely is full recovery. On the other hand, coincident sadness is associated with increased intensity and persistence.[65] So it is with neck pain. Fortunately, most alternative therapists are gentle when it comes to applying various modalities to the elderly neck. Unfortunately, spine surgeons know no such fears. The necks of Medicare beneficiaries are suffering the same fate as their low backs. Between 1992 and 2005, the rates of complex cervical fusions have more than doubled nationwide—tenfold in some places, like Boise, Idaho.[66] The commonest diagnosis offered as the rationale for all the cutting and fusing is "cervical spondylosis with myelopathy." "Cervical" means neck, and "spondylosis" is a fancy term for all the age-related changes in the bones of the spine.

"Myelopathy" is at the cutting edge. It denotes something wrong with the substance of central-nervous-system tissue; in the neck, that means the substance of the spinal cord itself. Cervical myelopathy is not a cause of neck pain. It is a neurologic disorder that affects the nerve connections as they course through the neck and on to their final destinations else-where down the body. In fact, cervical myelopathy characteristically af-fects the nerves that leave the spinal canal last. Therefore, the symptoms of cervical myelopathy are difficulty with gait and with bladder and bowel control. There are distinctive findings on neurological examination that help make this diagnosis so that when full blown, there is no doubt that the spinal cord in the neck is damaged. Cervical myelopathy is very rare. So how is it that we're witnessing rapid escalation of surgical procedures for a disease that is very rare?

This is spinal stenosis redux. Neck pain is very common. So, too, are the proclivity of American physicians to get imaging studies and the ex-pectation of the American patient to be studied and to receive a "you're normal" report. Degenerative changes of the cervical spine are ubiquitous and often impressive in magnitude, seeming to compress the spinal cord in the neck. Even these impressive images are common in well, asymp-tomatic people. Can these images be ignored in someone who has symp-toms of any sort? What happens if there are hints to trouble walking, or more urinary frequency than had been customary, or even a degree of in-continence? How can one assume that the image of a crushed spinal cord is an incidental finding? Shouldn't the pressing on the cord be relieved? And if that requires extensive surgery, once ripped asunder, shouldn't the spinal cord be stabilized with some widget or other?

I received a call from a friend in another city. He's one of the nation's leading attorneys who himself is approaching aged worker status. His wife is a few years younger and a vigorous, athletic woman — or she was before she developed neck pain. The attorney threw his weight around to get her an expedited appointment with the society spine surgeon of the city. She could not recall a detailed history having been taken, let alone a detailed neurological examination. She had neck pain, she got an MRI, she was told she had cervical myelopathy, and she was scheduled for surgery. I was called. I arranged for an examination by a thorough physician who could find no neurologic clues to myelopathy. We said, "No thank you," to the surgery. Her neck pain resolved in a month and she has been well for years. We don't know why she was hurting, but we wished it away despite the persistence of the bony overgrowth.

Interestingly, I am not certain spine surgery works for classic cervical myelopathy. The likelihood of a return of neurologic function is uncertain based on published clinical experiences and two attempts at systematic trials.[67] That is true also for "cauda equina syndrome," which is the rare case where something pushes into the spinal canal in the low back. The spinal cord actually ends near the bottom of the chest; the rest of the canal is occupied by a bundle of nerve roots that look like a horse's tail (a cauda equina). Pressing on the cauda equina also causes difficulties with bowel and bladder function and with sensation in the groin area. Cauda equina syndrome occurs when bony spurs, discal herniation, or other tissues extend into the spinal canal. Despite the uncertain outcome of extensive surgery for cervical myelopathy or cauda equina syndrome, most argue that the neurologic damage can be so debilitating it's worth the risk.[68] That risk/benefit assessment does not pertain to pain in the neck or in the low back without neurologic compromise at any age. As far as I'm concerned, operating on painfulness in the neck or low back of elderly people is unconscionable. But I never make the decision for my patient who is offered a surgical remedy. I am willing to offer my advice if asked. However, I never withhold a discussion of the science that might inform their decision making. Presenting this information is a primary responsibility of the physician in the twenty-first century. If the patient chooses a surgical option for spine pain, I stand by them fully and participate in the encouragement that facilitates their recovery.

Pinched Nerve

My reasoning regarding the surgical option for a "pinched nerve" parallels that for the painful spinal disorders just mentioned. The technical term for pain shooting down the arm or the leg is radiculopathy, which implies that something is irritating the root of the nerve as it exits the spine to innervate some part of the arm or leg. Radiculopathy can be very unpleasant. However, we are not certain of the actual cause at the site of the exiting root and not completely certain of which root is irritated, since there is considerable overlapping. Hence, the surgical option for radiculopathy is another crude hit-or-miss attempt to remove something in the neighborhood of the root that might be doing the irritating. Fortunately, whatever the something is, it tends to "heal" on its own; radiculopathy is nearly always self-limited. That means it goes away—the good news. The bad news is that it can take many months to do so. The scientific literature in the working-age population suggests that surgically mucking about may help in the short term but not in the long term, and the "price" of the short-term benefit is the grief of recovering from surgery and the risks of the procedures. In elderly persons, that price would be intolerable even if it purchased such a minor advantage.

Of course, radiculopathy can represent more than shooting pain; it can represent damage to the "pinched nerve," resulting in weakness. A neurological compromise such as demonstrable weakness puts me on thinner ice when it comes to a potential surgical remedy—as did cauda equina syndrome and classic cervical myelopathy. If it were me, I would forego the surgery for radiculopathy even in the face of weakness, which usually can be overcome since it affects only a particular muscle group and not the entire extremity. But that's me. When it's a patient who has to make this decision, I suggest a conference that allows him or her to ask pointed questions of me and the consulting surgeon. If we ever undertook a randomized sham-controlled trial of surgery for radiculopathy in elderly patients, we could truly inform, if not forewarn, the patient. I consider it unethical that we, all of us, are not demanding such.

I have been doing a lot of bashing of surgeons and their fellow travelers, from those who do violence to our coronary arteries to those who do violence to our spines. I don't find the euphemistic "they have a hammer" to be a defense for procedures that are effective in their "experience" but have only the most tenuous of scientific underpinning, if any. I would want us as a nation to stop underwriting an enterprise such as this, one that is at the margins of our community ethic or beyond. As far I'm concerned, and as I've stated repeatedly in the print, broadcast, and broadband media, nothing of this nature should be supported until there is robust scientific evidence for clinically meaningful benefit in some subset of eligible patients. Once we're sure there is benefit for pink zebras, then it is easy to seek benefit in green zebras. If we have no evidence that a procedure really works in any subset, then evidence that it "works as well" may be evidence that it works as poorly.

I will shortly sing the praises of orthopedic surgeons in the context of hip surgery, though not knee surgery. I need surgeons for the sake of my patients. And I respect "surgical judgment," which I define as the skill set they offer my patients once they are under anesthesia and in recovery. Surgical judgment for earlier generations related to diagnostic acumen and the a priori appraisal of surgical outcome (the judgment as to how much you will or will not be helped if you have the procedure). Today, the diagnostic acumen of surgeons has largely been co-opted by the exquisite advances in imaging and laboratory testing. Since surgeons are masters of the concrete (something they can see or feel), the absence of a demonstrable surgical target in the course of a modern diagnostic workup is largely determinative. The presence of the target should be less determinative; it should call for surgical judgment to say whether we should operate, wait, or forego the surgical option. Today, when the risks of procedures themselves are fewer and the payments for not operating pale next to the payments for operating, simply the presence of the target is usually sufficient.

This dialectic calls for wide recognition and aggressive reform. In the twenty-first century, when alternative options offer uncertain advantages, science — not payments — should be the mediator. Because I feel so strongly about that, I'm willing to advocate for, and explain the rationale for, sham-controlled procedure trials, just as we expect science to inform the licensing of pharmaceuticals. In the twenty-first century, patients are entitled to reliable information as the basis of rational decision making. Relying on the hubris of the practitioner is the fallback of the past. When it comes to neck pain, low back pain, pain moving a shoulder, and pain in a lower-extremity joint with weight bearing, "in my experience" doesn't cut it as a rationale for surgical intervention, even if the intervention is described as "minimally invasive" or the "arthroscopic" buzz word is brandished. There are orthopedists all over the country with an arthroscope at the ready to "fix" you — in every hamlet, in freestanding orthopedic surgical centers, in sports medicine centers, in occupational medicine centers, seemingly in every garage and in every pot. Furthermore, many of these orthopedists cluster, and many either own their "imaging center" or are in a similarly conflictual relationship with another's "imaging center." Many won't even see you without first putting you through the claustrophobic wizardry of an MRI study. Some can find reason for a CṪ ("CAT") scan, despite the inexcusable radiation exposure that is involved. Almost all of this activity satisfies my definition of Type II Medical Malpractice — doing the unnecessary, even if it is done well. Elective orthopedics is coauthoring the bleakest chapter in the history of Western medicine with the interventional cardiologists. Let me arm you with the information you need so that you and your primary-care physician can see clearly through the morass of hype and marketing. I have written extensively about this in my books aimed at the general audience and at the professional audience,[69] but in the context of the working-age adult. Here, I am focusing on the clinical challenges that relate to later life.

Upper-Extremity Challenges

There are two age-related processes that are ubiquitous and always challenging to comfort and function: disorders of the shoulder and hand osteoarthritis. Neither has escaped important and extensive scientific inquiry. The inferences that result would seem to be inescapable, but both the medical community and the general public have managed to escape from them.

Many older people, as many as 25 percent, are aware of a painful shoulder today.[70] There are many causes of shoulder pain, but we will consider only the form of shoulder pain that accounts for nearly all of this morbidity. This form afflicts one shoulder and has no traumatic precipitant. The onset can be relatively sudden, a matter of days, or it can sneak up over weeks. The shoulder is not particularly painful during the day as long as the arm is hanging at one's side, with the elbow bent or not. Some movement can be relatively pain free, such as putting one's hand in one's lap. But a motion such as trying to comb one's hair is painful and may be so painful as to be prohibitive. The shoulder may be tender to touch, sometimes very tender, but only at a particular spot, usually at the side of the shoulder. Uninterrupted sleep may be difficult, in large part because rolling over is painful. However, the shoulder is not warm and does not look different from before it started hurting or different from the other shoulder.

Shoulder pain is a common reason people seek medical attention. However, most people with shoulder pain do not consult their doctor and are no worse off for staying away.[71] I'm not sure how these folks manage. Maybe they rely more on the shoulder that isn't hurting. Regardless, they shoulder their burdens, put their shoulder to the wheel, and march on shoulder to shoulder until they are rewarded with spontaneous regression of the symptoms in the months ahead. The minority who seek care for shoulder discomfort is enriched with people for whom life is serving up other challenges, particularly psychosocial challenges.[72] This is true of back pain and many other complaints; in our society, it is far easier to consider the pain the primary problem rather than a surrogate complaint for the psychosocial challenge.

And Western physicians are trained only to hear about the pain in the shoulder and not everything else that is painful in the patient's life. Patient and doctor focus on what is wrong with the shoulder and what can be done about the disorder. Clearly, there is something going on with the very complex structure we call the shoulder joint. In addition to the main joint (the glenohumeral joint), there is another small joint nearby at the end of the clavicle. There are many muscles involved in shoulder motion, many about the joint and under the joint with tendons going every which way, including through the joint. The rotator cuff is a group of small muscles that surround the main joint and have a minor role in shoulder motion and stability. Most of the motion and stability is served by large muscles, not by the rotator cuff. Furthermore, the shoulder floats on the rib cage, so you can shrug and move the entire shoulder without moving the main joint itself. So what's hurting?

Truth be told, when it comes to the older patient, no one has the foggiest idea what's wrong with the shoulder that makes it hurt so. But that won't stop them from giving you a label: bursitis, periarthritis, tendonitis, or, horror of horrors, a rotator cuff tear. And this being modern medicine, you will be imaged with routine X-rays and often with an MRI. It is highly unlikely that the shoulder of an older person will prove any more pristine than does the spine. The joints themselves may be unimpressive, but not the tendons. We know from autopsy studies that a third of people over age sixty have complete tears through one or both rotator cuffs.[73] But the MRI is far more sensitive to changes in soft tissues such as the muscles and tendons about the shoulder, including the rotator cuff. For seventy-five years, orthopedists have been taught, and still teach, that the rotator cuff is subject to tears that can cause shoulder pain and can be surgically repaired if necessary.[74] No doubt there is some truth to this in young people, although I take issue with the belief in a surgical remedy. However, forget it for elderly people. For octogenarians, abnormalities of the cuff and of the edge of the main joint are the rule; they are normal findings, whether hurting or not. Not just for the elderly but for all comers with painful shoulders who have abnormal rotator cuffs on MRI, there is no relationship between the level of pain or disability and the location and size of full thickness tears. In fact, nothing seen in the muscles and tendons is specific for shoulder pain. Ascribing the form of shoulder pain we're discussing to any particular disorder of the older shoulder is sophistry.[75] And operating on any such disorder is the epitome of Type II Medical Malpractice. It makes no sense, and the track record in older patients is awful.

Surgery is out of the question if one is appropriately informed.[76] But that is not all that will be offered in nearly every general practice and certainly every orthopedic practice. There is a long-standing tradition of

injecting the tenderest spot on the shoulder with a corticosteroid preparation that dissolves very slowly. This never made much sense. Thanks to
many randomized placebo-controlled trials of injecting the hurting shoulder, another tradition can be relegated to the dustbin of history.[77] Maybe
there is some short-term benefit if the onset is sudden, but otherwise,
warm showers and over-the-counter analgesics do as well.

The other tradition that is sure to be offered is a referral to a physical
therapist. This tradition also dates back seventy-five years to the same
source, the Massachusetts General Hospital, where pioneering orthope-
dist Ernest Codman was formulating the notion of rotator cuff disease
that remains largely immutable to this day. Physical therapists go to great
lengths to help patients with shoulder pain improve their range of motion. One operating principle is that this is necessary to avoid a frozen
shoulder—an incorrect principle since "frozen shoulder" is a rare and
separate disease and not the result of progression from usual shoulder
pain. One study is particularly informative, a randomized controlled trial
of corticosteroid injection versus physiotherapy for persistent shoulder
pain.[78] There was no difference in outcome. However, before randomization, these subjects were asked if they had a preference in treatment.
Those who had a preference and were randomized to the treatment they
preferred did better than those who had no preference or were randomized to the treatment they didn't prefer. The mind is a wondrous thing.

If it were me, I'd join the majority of people with the usual shoulder
pain who deal on their own. If I wasn't sure this was the usual shoulder
pain, I'd ask my physician to opine, and if the consensus was "usual shoulder pain," I'd get on with life. If I couldn't get on with life, the conversa-
tion would not relate to the shoulder but to the impediments that made it
hard for me to get on with life despite the shoulder pain.

HAND PAIN

Osteoarthritis of the hands is the fate of all of us. All our joints are bio-
logically active. As is true for our bone, we systematically degrade and
restore the various components of our joints throughout life. When we're
young, this process is highly organized, and the replacement parts are as
pristine as the originals. As we age, we are progressively less efficient.
The replacement of cartilage is less robust, and bony spurs grow out of
the margins of the joints. These spurs are covered with healthy cartilage
but in a useless anatomical site. This degenerative process reflects an element of wear and tear. However, the influence of normal wear and tear

is surprisingly minor.[79] It's trivial for the spine and slight for the hands. The predisposition for disorganized repair is largely inherited. We need to expunge the "wear and tear" notion from our mindset. Blame mom or pop—or both—instead.

So hand osteoarthritis is ubiquitous, but the age of onset and the magnitude of involvement runs in families. Men and women are affected, but the onset in women is at least a decade sooner than in men. Furthermore, we are likely to be affected earlier in life than our parents. And hand problems after fifty are not to be trivialized. They are present in nearly half of elderly people during the course of the year. For elderly women and all who are very old, they challenge the quality of daily living.[80] Most of this relates to hand osteoarthritis, and much can be avoided.

Hand osteoarthritis is a lesson in the biological complexities of this genetically determined disorganized repair. Not all joints in the hand are involved. The wrist and the metacarpophalangeal (MCP) joints are spared. The MCP joints are at the base of the fingers and are critical for grip strength. However, the DIP and PIP joints are principal targets (Figure 8), resulting in deformity and rigidity, which can interfere with fine motions but does not severely compromise grip. All of us should take advantage of these biomechanical considerations long before we find our function compromised. So many tasks that customarily demand pincer movements can be done with grip, particularly if the task content is modified. Turning door knobs can be difficult if they are round, but opening with a lever handle presents no challenge. Tools, particularly writing and kitchen implements, with thick handles are far less challenging to use than those that demand pincer motions. And some tasks must be relearned; for example, picking up a purse or briefcase by gripping the handle instead of pinching it should become natural.

The other target of hand osteoarthritis that frequently causes problems is involvement of the first CMC joint (Figure 9-A). This joint anchors the thumb for powerful pinching motions. Osteoarthritis of the first CMC joint is usually pain free, but the joint can be tender for weeks at a time, during which pinching can be prohibitively painful. The "cure" is to avoid pinching. That's not so difficult once you reflect on the biomechanical alternatives. After all, gripping is still pain free, and many tasks that customarily invoke pinching can be accomplished by gripping. Figures 9-B and 9-C illustrate such a biomechanical adaptation.

There are other options. Intermittent use of low-dose, over-the-counter, anti-inflammatory drugs can take the sting out of the symptom-

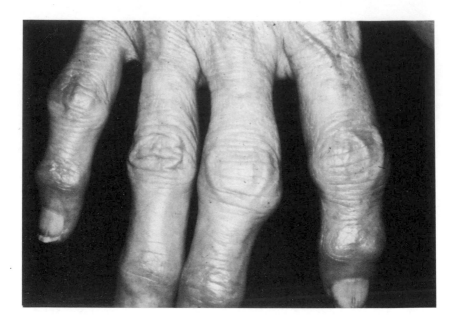

Figure 8. Characteristically, hand osteoarthritis first leads to the formation of bumps at the joints near the end of the fingers. These are the distal interphalangeal (DIP) joints, and the bumps are termed Heberden's nodes. Next to be similarly involved are the joints in the middle of the fingers, the proximal interphalangeal (PIP) joints, forming Bouchard's nodes. The joints at the base of the fingers, the metacarpophalangeal (MCP) joints, are spared. Joints with Heberden's and Bouchard's nodes are often misaligned and have restricted range of motion.

atic periods. Many are willing to inject the symptomatic first CMC joint with steroids; despite their preconceptions, they can accomplish only a fleeting placebo effect by doing so.[81] There are hand surgeons willing to remove the joint and replace it with a silicone spacer. That results in a painful, prolonged recovery and usually a good cosmetic outcome. As for function, the surgeons hem and haw as to prognosis, so why not stick with sensible biomechanical adaptations?

Lower-Extremity Challenges

A probability sample of the women over seventy residing in western Australia were asked how often they experienced lower-extremity pain on a five-point scale, with 1 equaling never, 2 equaling less than once a month, and so on up to 5 equaling once a day or more.[82] They were further asked where they hurt and whether pain led to consequences related to func-

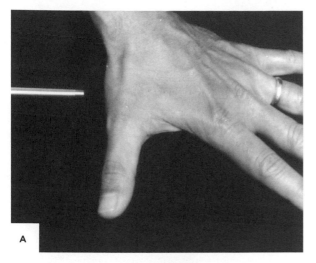

A

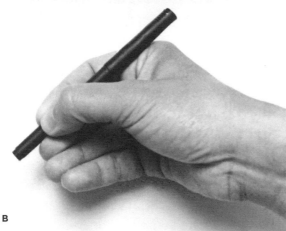

B

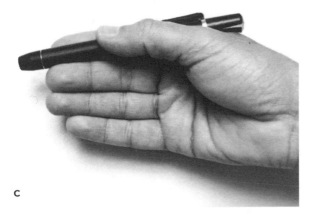

C

Figure 9. The aspect of hand osteoarthritis that can be most limiting is involvement of the first carpometacarpal (first CMC) joint. This is the joint at the base of the thumb. In Frame A, the pointer indicates the region of the first metacarpal, the bone that contributes to the formation of the first CMC joint at its base and the first MCP joint distally. Osteoarthritis of the first CMC joint can restrict its motion, so that spreading the thumb from the second digit is progressively limited. More important, the joint can be painful. Since it anchors the thumb, it is under most pressure in pinching forcefully. Hence, holding a writing instrument in pinch (Frame B) can be uncomfortable, whereas holding it along the length of the digits (Frame C) is not. Using a fat instrument facilitates the latter.

tion and quality of life. Only 28 percent said they never hurt. About 15 percent hurt in the hip, knee, and foot but not necessarily at the same time. The prevalence of women reporting any hip, knee, and foot pain was 39 percent, 52 percent, and 34 percent, respectively. Of course, the frequency of pain correlated with reduced mobility and quality of life. This is not a trivial problem, either. But it is not what it seems at first blush:

- Do not assume that because these joints hurt, they are damaged.
- Do not assume that whatever osteoarthritis is present is the cause of the joint pain.
- Do not assume that the joint pain is the cause of the compromise in mobility or quality of life.

Many people who have made these assumptions have been subjected to unnecessary procedures and pharmaceuticals. Some are no wiser, since they are "better" and unaware that they would have done as well without the interventions. Some are wiser because they are no better, and may be even worse off, for the intervening; but, as we have seen repeatedly in other contexts, these are wont to further assume that the reason for the dismal outcome was the magnitude of their disease, not the ineffectiveness and hazardous nature of the intervention.

There are instances when a surgical option is compelling and tempered only by considerations that relate to the surgical insult, not the surgical indication. Many procedures at the lower extremity are "major" surgery. All are "elective" in the sense that they are designed to maintain mobility—but not at all cost. A successful total hip replacement is less successful if the patient doesn't survive the procedure at all or lives only for a short time afterward. As a corollary, the "benefit" one seeks primarily relates to mobility and pari passu the severity of biomechanical compromise. "Pain," including pain with weight bearing that impedes mobility, is not a compelling indication for surgery.

Experienced surgeons know the truth in the last statement. They learned it the hard way. Every time a lower-extremity orthopedic surgeon evaluates a patient with a painful hip or knee or ankle or foot, there is a conflict between this statement and hubris in the form of, "I know the cause and I am capable of fixing it." This is not a level playing field. The surgeon is predisposed to operate because that is what surgeons are trained to do and are rewarded for doing. Furthermore, orthopedic and podiatric surgeons have a bag of tricks for pummeling whatever anatomical abnormality they deem to be causing the pain. New tricks are purveyed all the time. Remember, these are "devices" that are licensed by the FDA without a prerequisite for the demonstration of long-term efficacy. Remember, also, that these various devices are marketed to surgeons with an aggressiveness that always walks a fine ethical line and has been known to cross over to the illegal on more than one occasion. Financial incentives and conflicts of interest abound.

The usual surgeon/patient discussion plays out as follows. Some anatomical cause for the principal symptom is postulated, an abnormality that has been demonstrated on radiographs or by an MRI. Always there is a procedure that is designed to alter the anatomical abnormality in a way that is said to be beneficial. Seldom is there a rush to surgery. Rather, the surgeon is trained to advise "conservative" therapy first: analgesics, anti-inflammatory drugs, self-directed exercises, water aerobics, formal physical therapy, and the like. But the implication of "conservative" varies from wimpy to waste of time in the surgeon's demeanor, the patient's preconceptions, the popular press, and the public's mindset. A real American would want the damn thing fixed. "Conservative" is doomed to fail more often than not when such is the preconception. And "failed conservative therapy" is the leading indication for lower-extremity joint surgery.

I have long been fascinated by the evolution in the notions of "conservative" and "aggressive." At mid-twentieth century, when evidence-based medicine was in its infancy, "do no harm" was the ethical standard and "conservative" a good thing. "Aggressive" was the imprecation for doing the unaccepted; it lived on the borders of quackery and malpractice. In the 1960s, anesthesiology and postoperative care blossomed. Before then, anesthesia was administered by dripping ether on a gauze pad held over the face. Since then, it is delivered by tubes inserted into the windpipe by anesthetists who command technological gadgetry designed to get us through the procedure unscathed. And antibiotics and other drugs get us through the recovery period. Without these advances that relate to the surgical process, operating on the heart of a frail patient was exceedingly hazardous and largely prohibitive. It became routine, so routine that CABG surgery took hold, bringing with it the notion that "aggressive" was good and "conservative" nihilistic. The result is that "Can do?" has superseded "Should do?" in elective surgical decision making.

When it comes to lower-extremity joint surgery, there are few firm and fixed guidelines for the decision to have a procedure. The degree of osteoarthritis is a relative indication. That's because there is a remarkable degree of discordance between symptoms at a weight-bearing joint and radiographic damage. I pointed this out in an editorial twenty years ago.[83] It is particularly true for hip disease, where even the biomechanical compromise can be circumvented, particularly if the involvement is unilateral. It is true of forefoot disease, too. Knee pain is intermittent in all people but more frequent and more severe in people with the most severely osteoarthritic knees. It is intermittent nonetheless in any individual patient,[84] even with severe involvement. With time and support, particularly supportive communities, a remarkable number of people who are deemed surgical candidates for hip or knee surgery find that they no longer "need" the procedure. That was true in the past for about a third of the patients on a Canadian "wait list" for hip surgery and for elderly women waiting for knee surgery in a New York orthopedic hospital.[85] Today, the conveyor belt to the operating room is more efficient.

NONOPERATIVE THERAPY

How can it be that an osteoarthritic weight-bearing joint can be painful enough to bring one to a surgeon and then become less painful without a change in radiographs or MRI? We are not certain, but two influences are in play. First, something in the joint hurts. There are studies that suggest that this something is a small change in the bony structure underlying the joint — think microfractures that can heal. But then there's the lesson of Mrs. K.'s vertebroplasty that introduced this chapter. Superimposed on the pain is all the anticipatory anxiety and compromise in function. Coping with this insult is a demanding exercise that can easily be thwarted by confounders in life, such as loneliness or lack of social support in general. It is also confounded by being overweight, as we discussed in chapter 3. Extra girth is adding demand to weight-bearing joints with each step and rendering the painful joint even more painful. Interestingly, while extra weight has some association with the development of osteoarthritic damage of the knee, it has little if any relationship to progression.[86] That brings us to another of the mysteries of osteoarthritis. We've learned about genetic predisposition at the spine, hands, and knees, but each particular joint has its own set of predisposing factors. That's obvious when one realizes that hip and knee osteoarthritis is common, but seldom in the same person, and no one gets osteoarthritis of the true ankle joint.

Seeking medical attention is driven more by confounded coping than by pain or biomechanical compromise. Anything that diminishes confounding to coping is at least as therapeutic as other aspects of "conservative" therapy: exercising with a peer group, physical therapists more for their psychological support than the specifics of physical therapy, talk therapists regarding loneliness, and so forth. I am long convinced that the advantaged elderly who have access to water- or land-based[87] programs under the rubric "arthritis" are helped not simply because of the benefits of muscle building, but because of the benefits of peer support and interactions.

Of course, no one has joint pain without running into over-the-counter (OTC) and prescription remedies. Regarding the former, the occasional nonsteroidal anti-inflammatory is probably safe in the elderly, certainly safe enough for the FDA to approve many for OTC sales. I advise against any use of this class of agents in the elderly for regional musculoskeletal symptoms, including symptoms at weight-bearing joints. Peptic ulcer disease is most common in the elderly and most likely to be asymptomatic—until OTC nonsteroidal anti-inflammatory agents such as Aleve, Motrin, or aspirin stir them up so that they bleed. That is not a risk with acetaminophen, which is as effective (or ineffective) in palliating painful weight-bearing joints and, in intermittent low doses, quite safe. There is no data supporting the marketing that suggest that any prescription nonsteroidal anti-inflammatory agent is safer or more effective than the OTC members of this class of drugs. Therefore, prescription nonsteroidal anti-inflammatory drugs are no more appealing an option then their OTC cousins.

In May 2009 the American Geriatrics Society issued a revised guideline for the pharmacologic management of nonmalignant pain in elderly patients. They have come to share my concerns about nonsteroidal anti-inflammatories, although for the wrong reasons. They are more concerned about cardiovascular toxicities, which are particularly important in patients with heart failure[88] but not as frequent as gastrointestinal toxicity in all comers. They are in accord with my recommending acetaminophen as the analgesic of first choice. They had shared my antipathy toward opiates in a 2002 guideline, but they reversed themselves in the May 2009 revision. The reversal is testimony to the fashion in which marketing of opiates and the "pain lobby" have influenced the American zeal for squelching pain at all cost. I will stand my ground. Most of the conditions at the root of the nonmalignant pain that the elderly face are captured in this chapter. Always there are options for management that focus on coping and adaptation that can diminish the associated suffering, after which opiate treatment is seldom necessary. Furthermore, there is a hefty price that opiates place on the elderly beyond the obligate severe constipation: blunted sensorium, delirium, falls and fractures, urinary difficulties, and much more. I am not alone in decrying the use of opiates to palliate regional musculoskeletal symptoms in the elderly[89] or in any other age group.[90]

There are industries that live off of nonsurgical modalities marketed to improve symptoms in weight-bearing joints. It's your money, but realize how poorly so many of these options fare when studied systematically. Acupuncture,[91] therapeutic ultrasound,[92] and joint lavage[93] (washing out the joint) are expensive and time-consuming ways to get a placebo effect. Studies of injecting the joints with steroids or joint constituents (hyaluron preparations) yield varying results but never dramatic or long-term benefit. Maybe if a radiologist injects a symptomatic osteoarthritic hip with steroids, one can anticipate a bit more benefit,[94] but I doubt that will hold up any better than all the other encouraging results. As far as I'm concerned, various minerals and neutraceuticals, including glucosamine, are a waste of money; there have been numerous trials with variable results but never impressive outcomes for peripheral joints or back pain.[95]

In addition to attention to muscle strength, weight loss, and attitude, there are ways to adapt the architecture of the living space to accommodate biomechanical compromise in the weight-bearing joints. Elevating chair and toilette height can significantly reduce the challenges of knee disease. Avoiding stairs, either by circumvention or lifts, can help as well; knee diseases make descending difficult and risky, whereas ascending is the nemesis for those with hip osteoarthritis. Canes can improve balance, self-confidence, and safety from falling.

And, for some, there is a surgical solution.

OPERATIVE THERAPY

Hip, knee, and forefoot surgery requires skill and experience. I'm not sure it's the highest form of sculpture, but it has much in common, down to the chisels and hammers. You want a surgeon with a track record either to do your surgery or supervise whoever is chiseling away. You want to be very cautious about any surgeon who offers the latest design of widget she wants to put into your joint. Remember that these devices are not required to have any long-term record of safety and durability before being placed in your body. Remember that widgetry is a viciously competitive marketplace with all kinds of hidden agendas. Stick with the tried and true.

Surgery for osteoarthritis of the hip. The hip is a remarkably well-designed joint. It is a glistening ball-in-socket joint with an impressive range of motion limited by powerful muscles and an extraordinarily strong capsule, which makes the joint inherently stable. Osteoarthritis attacks the ball, which loses its smooth, elastic cartilage cap and becomes rough and irregular and somehow induces similar changes in the cup. There were many attempts at a surgical remedy during the first half of the twentieth century, but all were disappointing. The modern age of hip-replacement surgery began with the magnificent contribution of the late Sir John Charnley. Working in a provincial hospital near the Welsh border, Charnley built brilliantly on the work of earlier surgeons. He borrowed the idea of a stainless-steel replacement for the ball part of the joint, a small ball on a long metallic stem, from Austin Moore at Johns Hopkins, who introduced it to replace only that part of the joint when it was fractured. He fashioned a high-molecular-weight polyethylene cup, which he screwed into the socket. And he used an acrylic glue to attach components he couldn't screw to the bone. Charnley's genius was to remove the entire old joint, saw the ball part off the femur and gouge out the old cup, and replace it with new components. It healed, had a low-friction pivot, and regained stability, thanks to the power of the surrounding muscles. It was the greatest accomplishment of orthopedics in the twentieth century. Charnley's design has dominated since the 1970s; alternatives are introduced with great trepidation. Some have proved their worth. All truly remove the old hip, and in so doing all the nerves, to that region. That explains why the postoperative course is usually quite benign and rehabilitation efficient; without a nerve supply, the new hip is pain free.

Nancy Lane has said: "The optimal time to perform total hip replacement in patients with osteoarthritis is uncertain."[96] But the procedure is so successful, and rehabilitation so well tolerated, that the proclivities of all involved are to go sooner rather than later. However, it is still major surgery, with all the attendant potential for complications. There are also long-term complications. And it's not always so successful. To find this out, someone other than the operating surgeon or those involved with the operating surgeon has to ask patients how they are doing following any procedure. Since surgery is such a dramatic life event, we are predisposed to find the results "good" or better particularly when we're trying to please our surgeon. When others ask in confidence, perhaps a quarter of patients have important hip symptoms in the long term, and half of those are not better off for the surgery.[97] That's sobering. Couple that with the earlier experience in Canada: about a third of patients awaiting hip replacement decide they no longer need it when their number comes up. So it's as good a procedure as we can get, but not good enough to leap for it without a great deal of forethought and a wise physician to inform the fore thinking.

Surgery for knee osteoarthritis. It's easy to find people coping with knee pain today. And it's easy to find people whose knee X-rays have some degree, or even a great amount, of osteoarthritic changes. Over age sixty, it's even easier, and by age eighty, it's a dime a dozen. Only a fraction at any age has both knee pain and knee osteoarthritis at the same time, and many will become asymptomatic on their own if given the chance. One reason for the discordance between symptoms and osteoarthritic changes is that the knee is a complex joint with three distinct compartments that seem to have their own rules. Furthermore, some of the osteoarthritic changes are not always bad for you. For example, those whose lifestyle included much weight-bearing activities are more likely to have spurs around the joint but healthier cartilage in the joint. These spurs are no different from the spurs that accompany the destruction of the cartilage in other people. We think of the spurs that occur in the setting of good cartilage to be a healthy response to usage, whereas in the setting of osteoarthritic cartilage, they are a vain attempt at repair. Epidemiologists have long been aware of the demanding nature of defining "osteoarthritis."[98] If one includes "any knee pain ever" in someone with any osteoarthritic change, one can generate an inference that nearly half of people will qualify for the label at some point in their lifetime.[99] Numbers such as these may tickle the fancy of fund-raisers, marketers needing to sensationalize, and maybe policy makers. But they should serve as a forewarning to clinicians, particularly surgeons, and to their patients. How certain are you that my knee pain can be ascribed to the particular structural abnormality that is detected?

My approach to this conundrum, as you might guess, is to err toward the conservative. I am very cautious about leaping to a causal association with any osteoarthritic anatomical change and any symptom at the knee (and many other sites, such as the spine). I am less cautious in the setting of advanced osteoarthritis, where the intrinsic stability of the knee is compromised so that mobility and stability are challenged. Unlike the hip, the knee is not an inherently stable joint. It is essentially two platforms that hinge in bending with nothing solid holding them together, as opposed to the hip, where the ball fits snugly into its socket and is held there by powerful ligaments. The ligaments in the knee (the cruciates) and around the knee (the menisci and collaterals) are not so powerful and are often found to have torn in people with no knee symptoms. The platforms are held together by the orchestration of the function of the muscles of the thigh and calf, whose tendons course in front of and behind the knee. When the platforms lose their cartilaginous buffers because of osteoarthritis (and usually unevenly), the biomechanics of the knee are compromised. Pain serves to further compromise biomechanics. The only solution is a total knee replacement. But a "total knee replacement" is a misnomer for the modern procedure, which is a resurfacing and realignment of the compartments. Early on, there were attempts to do a procedure similar to the total hip replacement (the knee was sawed out and replaced with a metal hinge), but the results were dismal. The resurfacing procedure has a much better track record. However, it is very demanding of surgical skillfulness, requiring a lot of experience. There are a good deal of entrepreneurial shenanigans going on with the bits and pieces used to resurface the compartments. Since the "total knee replacement" is not inherently stable, recovery is painful and prolonged, demanding great perseverance in regaining the muscle strength necessary for adequate biomechanics. There is plenty of opportunity for things to go awry along the way, especially in the older patient. And honest, long-term follow-up demonstrates far more dissatisfaction than with total hip replacements in the same age groups. This procedure is no walk in the park; Jane Brody of the *New York Times* and Don Berwick, director of the Center for Medicare and Medicaid Services, have published personal narratives that testify to that fact.

The efforts to fashion a better total knee replacement have percolated along for fifty years. The slow progress has stimulated many to think of ways to treat knee osteoarthritis earlier and perhaps impede its progression in the few for whom progression is likely to prove bitter. Enter the arthroscope. The rallying cry of modern surgeons is "minimally invasive surgery." That often translates into slipping tubes into the body through which video monitors can be connected, followed by surgical instruments that can snare or cut or burn or drill or whatever. Doing this to the knee was particularly appealing given the accessibility and the fact that there are no structures that can get in the way (like bowel or blood vessels). So getting there was straightforward; what you do once you get there was not so straightforward. My orthopedic colleagues came up with all sorts of great ideas for violence to do to the knee once they got inside. America loves the idea of minimally invasive, high-tech surgery for its own sake. After all, if it's minimally invasive and high tech—and covered by insurance—one assumes it must be effective. It rapidly became open season on the American knee, including the osteoarthritic knee of the older adult. The zeal for doing violence to knees (and shoulders of late) is unabated. It's unabated in spite of the science.

Science has tested the hypothesis that doing some sort of violence to the knee joint advantages the joint and therefore the person attached to it. J. Bruce Moseley and his colleagues[100] had the courage to do the testing despite knowing that if the result was unfavorable, the wrath of the orthopedic establishment would be their fate. They tested with a sham-controlled trial. A total of 180 patients with osteoarthritis of the knee were randomly assigned to receive arthroscopic débridement, arthroscopic lavage, or placebo surgery. Patients in the placebo group received skin incisions and underwent a simulated débridement without insertion of the arthroscope. Patients and assessors of outcome were blinded to the treatment-group assignment. Outcomes were assessed at multiple points over a twenty-four-month period with the use of five self-reported scores — three on scales for pain and two on scales for function — and one objective test of walking and stair climbing. At no point did either of the intervention groups report less pain or better function than the placebo group.

The response from the orthopedic establishment was predictable. They do the procedures differently, and they see patients quite different from the elderly male veterans at the Houston Veterans Administration Hospital. Arthroscopic procedures continued as the standard of care for elderly patients with symptomatic osteoarthritis.

In Canada, the belief that surgeons are the answer for knee pain is not as firmly held as it is in the United States. That's why the Canadians could design a randomized controlled trial comparing arthroscopic surgery for osteoarthritis of the knee with physical and medical therapy and have no crossovers — meaning that all those assigned to conservative care stayed there without demanding the surgery. Such a trial would not fly in the United States on scientific grounds because of crossovers and the likelihood of a surgery-related placebo effect. But the Canadian trial, published in 2008, is hard to ignore.[101] Arthroscopic surgery provided no additional benefit to optimized conservative therapy. An editorial by Robert Marx, an orthopedic surgeon on the staff of Cornell's prestigious Hospital for Special Surgery, accompanied this paper in the New England Journal of Medicine.[102] Marx argues that osteoarthritis is not the only cause of pain in the osteoarthritic knee and "arthroscopic surgery remains appropriate in patients with arthritis in specific situations."

Not to my way of thinking.

Bunions and more. Pristine, beautiful feet are youthful memories. After sixty-five, the vast majority of us have "foot issues." When asked, a random sample of nearly 800 residents of Smithfield, Massachusetts, aged sixty-five or older frequently reported toenail disorders (75 percent) and corns and calluses (60 percent), and a third had bunions. Toenail conditions were more common in men and bunions, corns, and calluses in women.[103] Nearly all these particular conditions in nearly all people of similar age nearly all the time do not associate with foot pain or interfere with gait.[104] That is not to say that disorders of the feet are purely cosmetic. In a survey of community-dwelling Australian adults over age seventy, a third were found on examination to have had "disabling foot pain" by criteria that included pain intensity, functional limitation, concern about appearance, and activity restriction. However, nearly all who exhibited these attributes also had elements of depression, flatter feet, and pain in other body regions.[105] Hence, the symptom of foot pain is often part of the more general experience I'm calling decrepitude.

Nonetheless, one needs to consider whether addressing foot issues themselves would advantage these elderly persons. There is a subset, about 10 percent, in surveys such as these that have chronic and more severe foot pain. These tend to be women, younger women closer to sixty-five than eighty-five and particularly those who were obese and had coincident hand or knee osteoarthritis.[106] Deciding which foot disorder is contributing to these symptoms in a given patient is not simple. Sometimes there is something obvious, such as a tender corn, that can be readily and effectively extirpated by someone skilled in doing so, usually a podiatrist. Sometimes there is important cracking and irritation between the toes than can respond to an OTC fungicidal cream. But most disorders of the skin and nails are annoying rather than painful and disabling.

Is the same true for bunions? Bunions (Figure 10) are not simply cosmetic deformities; they distort gait patterns in a fashion that could contribute to instability and a propensity to fall.[107] There is no doubt they are irritating as symbols of aging, and if one is not careful to purchase footwear with a wide "box" (the part where the toes are), they are easily irritated. One of my patients presented me with an antique implement that was inserted into the box of the shoe in the nineteenth century to punch a hole that accommodated the bunion. Today, one can usually find a "walking" shoe that accomplishes as much. Of course, there is a wealth of purveyors of shoes and shoe inserts (orthotics) marketed to salve whatever symptoms one is ascribing to their bunion or other regional musculo-

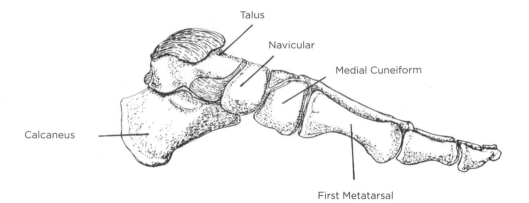

Talus

Navicular

Medial Cuneiform

Calcaneus

First Metatarsal

Figure 10. The big toe joint at the base of the first metatarsal bone is the first metatarsophalangeal (MTP) joint. A "bunion" is a severely osteoarthritic first MTP: the cartilage is lost; spurs form, most prominently at the inner margins of the joint; and the joint loses stability. Given the forces involved in gait, the big toe (the hallux) is pushed toward the outside (valgus), which makes the spurs more prominent and creates the hallux valgus, or bunion, deformity.

skeletal foot disorder. Systematic studies seeking meaningful benefit for orthotics are lacking in scientific rigor but not at all encouraging.[108]

As you might have guessed or known all too well, if there's a bony bump and an associated symptom, it's hard for any person not to associate one with the other, especially any person with the skills and proclivity for removing the putatively offending bump. Bunions are low-hanging bumps. Until recently, orthopedists had bigger bumps to violate. But now orthopedists have joined podiatrists in the assault on the bumps. I have always been concerned about the rationale for removing the bump since the osteoarthritic joint is left behind, as are the forces in gait that continue to test it. Removing and then fusing the first MTP (Figure 10) is substituting one disorder, a rigid big toe (hallux rigidus), for a bunion (hallux valgus). I remain very skeptical, despite a randomized controlled trial from Finland comparing surgery for moderately severe hallux valgus with orthotics or with "watchful waiting."[109] At twelve months, those who had the surgery had less pain and less trouble with footwear, though there was no difference in cosmetic concerns. These subjects were relatively young (mean age forty-eight) women. I'm not at all sure this result pertains to elderly persons, nor am I confident that these younger women won't come to regret the surgery twenty years later. But that's a reflection of my "first, do no harm" philosophy.

Besides, we may be doing violence to a result—a bunion—and ignoring its cause. There are many factors at play. One is genetic predisposition; the likelihood of bunion formation correlates with the age of onset and progression of hand osteoarthritis, which has an enormous genetic component and similar gender bias. However, while the onset and progression of hand osteoarthritis is measurably influenced by patterns of usage over time, osteoarthritis of the first MTP is greatly influenced by local forces. But that's not all. Most people with the more severe bunion deformities are flat-footed. If one looks closely, their ankles tend to be deformed, so that the heel is pushed outwards with heel strike. The configuration creates an abnormal set of forces, each promoting the next: heel pushed out, flattened midfoot, and big toe pushed out. In the normal foot, there is a tendon that starts from a powerful leg muscle and travels beneath the inside ankle bone (medial malleolus) to insert into the arch. This tendon, the tibialis posterior tendon, pulls up the arch and maintains normal alignment. If this mechanism goes awry, the flatfoot-bunion complex results. Unfortunately, once this has been established, the surgical remedy is unappealingly aggressive.[110] There are no studies, but maybe the next generation will be benefited in the long term by the popularity of shoes designed with biomechanical principles in mind.

6

FRAILTY

The etymology of the word "frailty" is telling. It derives from the Latin *fragilis*, to denote weakness, as in vulnerability. It could apply to an economy as much as to a sickly individual. It was adopted in the late twentieth century by the gerontology community as a syndrome diagnosis. To be old and frail was not simply the antithesis of being old and vigorous. Frailty was not the *result* of the accumulation of pathologies—weak bones, weak mind, weak muscles, and weak constitution. Frailty was the accumulation. Hence, frailty is a disease one can suffer on the far end of the continuum of disease states that underlies the transition from independence to dependence.[1] By this conceptualization, the frail elderly are at a way station before death. They are Oliver Wendell Holmes's Deacon's Masterpiece, the "One-Hoss Shay" at the end of its serviceable life, beleaguered by metal fatigue in each of its parts and destined to crumble. Maybe something can be done, some patchwork, but basically life has beaten the elderly person to frailty. The charges to medicine are to learn how to prevent frailty or to define the mechanism for the terrible process and halt it.

This is a conceptualization that has never rested easily with me. I view frailty as an existential state. It is a stage of life that has its peculiar attributes, some appealing and some unappealing. It offers up challenges for the person who is frail and for those who know that person. It also offers up rewards. I could describe raising a toddler, or being a teenager, or young married life and more in the same fashion. However, there are three attributes that make frailty unique among life's stages:

- The loss of any sense of invincibility
- The loss of competence in performing essential activities of daily living
- The realization that no life stage will supersede this one

Many who are not so old but are faced with progressive or terminal diseases qualify as frail. Many of the principles I will develop regarding frail elderly people pertain to all frail people, but the context for this chapter is the frail elderly person. The goal of the chapter is to reframe the notion of frailty as a stage of life that has positive, even joyful features for the frail elderly person and for those whose lives are touched by the frail elderly person. Society has no difficulty framing the precedent stage as the Golden Years. We all readily grasp the need to keep decrepitude a challenge rather than a lifestyle. It's not so easy with frailty. No one looks forward to frailty, but that does not mean that it's all so bad. True, it is a stage that is limited by the process of dying, but the process of dying and frailty are not the same. The process of dying has its own rules that commandeer the experience and that will occupy us in the next chapter. Frailty countenances elements of choice and a degree of resilience. Frailty is not the process of dying until it precludes relationship. As Martin Buber, in his book *I and Thou* (1923), described it:

> The You encounters me by grace — it cannot be found by seeking. But that I speak the basic word to it is a deed of my whole being, is my essential deed.
>
> The You encounters me. But I enter into a direct relationship to it. This the relationship is election and electing, passive and active at once. . . .
>
> The basic word I-You can be spoken only with one's whole being. The concentration and fusion into a whole being can never be accomplished by me, can never be accomplished without me. I require a You to become; becoming I, I say You.
>
> All life is encounter.

Frailty needs to be reframed in this light.

Vulnerability

The first element of frailty, the loss of a sense of invincibility, is reality based. It takes very little to topple the frail elderly person into the process of dying. And once in that vortex, there is little biological reserve to mobilize for reversal. Health care is high on the list of avoidable hazards.[2] This is true for all of us; I have written three books about medicalization and overtreatment in working-aged adults.[3] But elderly persons, and frail elderly persons in particular, are far more susceptible to adverse effects of health care. They are more likely to experience adverse effects of pharmaceuticals even at lower doses. Nonetheless, this is the most medicated population;[4] nearly all take at least one prescription drug, and about 40 percent of elderly people over age seventy-five take five or more prescription drugs. Furthermore, nearly half are also taking over-the-counter agents and assorted dietary supplements.

Too often all of this medicating goes on with inadequate monitoring for effectiveness and for toxicities.[5] Adverse effects of many drugs, including many commonly prescribed drugs, are frequent at all ages but far more likely to be catastrophic in the frail elderly.[6] An adverse effect such as grogginess can lead to a fall at any age, but a fall can lead to a fracture in the frail elderly from which recovery is less predictable. Even an uncomplicated wrist fracture can mark the onset of rapid decline.[7] Younger people are far more likely to recover from a complication such as intestinal bleeding than the frail elderly. All of this is ever more tragic since so many medicines prescribed for the elderly target long-term risks and hazards rather than active illness.[8] Treating octogenarians with agents that might offer someone some long-term benefit is an example of bad clinical judgment. Adverse consequences cannot be dismissed on benefit-risk grounds as there is no possibility of benefit. Such adverse consequences are examples of iatrogenicity, or diseases caused by the physician.

Underlying the medicalization and overtreatment of the elderly is a new kind of ageism in medicine. Traditionally, ageism was a term to denote the fashion in which older patients were ignored or undertreated. It remains a tension in a national health scheme such as Britain's,[9] in which finite moneys are allocated after considerations of costliness of interventions and their effectiveness. For British health policy, the fact that the elderly have fewer years remaining prejudices against underwriting costly interventions for them. In the United States, all sorts of stakeholders pressure the Centers for Medicare and Medicaid Services (CMS), which administers Medicare, with "we don't ration." The public has learned this mantra. As a result, cost-effectiveness has been expunged from considerations of indemnification, explicitly in the recent reform legislation.[10] Medicare might tweak the reimbursement schedules, but if it is in "common practice," it is paid for in the elderly. The result is a peculiarly American form of ageism. The elderly are afforded anything "approved" that money can buy, even if it affords them no health benefit and places them in harm's way. But the elderly are less likely to be afforded less-costly and less-profitable interventions. The reimbursement schedules caring about them as people and caring for them as patients pale next to reimbursement schedules for interventions aimed at their diseases. Cognitive care, such as informing medical decisions or planning for the future or even productive empathy, gets very short shrift in America.

All of these ramifications of the first element of frailty—the loss of a sense of invincibility—are not generally appreciated. They should be waved in the face of CMS administrators and all else who are involved in the care of frail elderly persons, whether paid or unpaid. Whenever possible, medical decisions should be made by frail elderly people themselves, only after they are fully informed as to the potential for benefit and the likelihood of harm. The same holds for anyone who has been designated to help make these decisions or to make them on behalf of the frail elderly person. The frail elderly is a population for which the phrase "less is more"[11] is much more likely to be a rational and compassionate therapeutic posture than ageism. Engaging the frail elderly in such decision making is part of honoring your father and mother.

Disability

The second aspect of frailty is the loss of competence to perform essential activities of daily living. Such disability is the usual focus of discussions of frailty and has driven a great deal of productive research that seeks ways to postpone or reduce disability. Progress has been apparent,[12] although much of this may simply reflect the demographic shifts in longevity discussed in chapter 1. "Progress" reflects the fact that we are living longer and therefore experience frailty later. However, some of the progress clearly reflects medical advances that are applied earlier in life. Cataract extraction with lens implantation is an example. Still, much that disables the elderly and contributes to frailty has no such ready solution. In elderly persons living in the community, functional status decline is multifactorial; cognitive impairment, depression, comorbid conditions, reduced physical capacity or activity, and low frequency of social contacts are among the critical elements.[13]

Physical frailty assaults a range of abilities. Some physical impairments are more disabling than others because they reflect the degree to which frailty has become global rather than because they preclude particular tasks. Sometimes, but not always, these are the same impairments. We learned this in studies that we undertook at UNC on the relationship between the upper-extremity physical capacity of community-dwelling elderly women and the likelihood they would maintain independent living.[14] We presented a sample of women with a panel of manual tasks that they were all able to complete. We then asked them to complete the tasks as rapidly as they could. The longer they took, the more likely they would require assisted living in the months to come. This result was not a reflection of any demonstrable neuromuscular disorder or other comorbid condition, nor could it be explained by effects of their medicines or the nature of their social networks. The physical impairment we demonstrated did not produce a limiting disability. It must be a surrogate measure of the degree of frailty. A similar observation has been made using the time to walk a long corridor as the performance measure; the longer it took, the sooner the elderly person died.[15] The corollary observation is that increasing and maintaining the level of physical activity of sedentary elderly increases the longevity only of less frail women.[16]

However, supervised, encouraged, and appropriate low-intensity exercises targeted at the relevant incapacities can retard progression of disability in frail elderly persons.[17] Remember, we are considering frailty in this chapter. In previous chapters, we were considering the advantages of exercise and of peer interactions for maintaining function before arriving at frailty. These advantages allow one to enter frailty with "a leg up." Once frail, exercise has different content and offers different advantages. Frail elderly persons may not have the physical capacity for more than low-intensity exercising and may not have the support system to pursue such activities anywhere but at home.

Low-intensity targeted exercises are the best we can do in terms improving physical ability. There is much more to be done in reducing physical demands. Attention to room and furniture configuration, adaptive and assistive devices, and the need for help can remarkably reduce disability and greatly enhance independence.

Depression in the frail elderly is common, often multifactorial, and more often mismanaged. It is one of many reasons that every elderly person should have established a therapeutic relationship with a wise physician long before arriving at frailty. Many medicines and a number of treatable medical conditions can cause depression; the former should have been thwarted at the outset and the latter treated proactively. No wise physician leaps to treating an elderly, let alone a frail elderly, depressed patient with pharmaceuticals. First, many of these drugs are dangerous in the elderly; the FDA has been strident in its warnings in that regard.[18] Second, antidepressants have a very unfavorable benefit-risk ratio for mild, moderate, or situational depressions in all patients,[19] particularly in the elderly. Too many people and patients and physicians have been fooled to think otherwise by egregious marketing schemes that take advantage of unconscionable shenanigans with the data.[20]

There has been a resurgence of various forms of behavioral and talk therapies that are starting to supplant all these pills. There are even randomized trials comparing such therapies with usual care that demonstrate benefit for anxiety disorders among older adults[21] and even insomnia.[22] The trend and its promise are very encouraging. What's missing is a commitment on the part of society to expend monies to underwrite the training and consultations of therapists rather than to pay for pills. Valuing the quality of life of frail elderly persons in this fashion requires the general realization that pills are expedient but do much more for purveyors than for patients.

URINARY INCONTINENCE
AND OTHER ASSAULTS ON DIGNITY

Rethinking Aging is not a textbook of geriatrics for the lay reader. I am choosing particular topics because they are object lessons designed to teach the reader why he or she should demand information that allows for informed medical decision making. Much that is awful can and often does befall the frail elderly. Some of it transitions to the next chapter and the process of dying. Some of it is amenable to medical treatments. There is a science that informs all these decision nodes. When the science is incomplete, the discussion relates to the level of uncertainty. The fallback is the "clinical judgment" of a wise physician.

Many of the insults to the quality of life of the frail elderly are inherent to frailty. Many, such as disability and depression, can be mollified with attention to the circumstance rather than attempting to treat the disease. Pelvic floor disorders are another example of a set of diseases that are best managed conservatively in the frail elderly woman. Pelvic floor disorders affect a substantial proportion of women and increase in prevalence with age to afflict over half of female octogenarians.[23] These disorders include urinary and/or fecal incontinence and prolapse (protrusion) of pelvic organs. Most women have learned to manage this on their own, mainly by dealing with embarrassment, stigmatization, and the expense of routine care products as best they can. For some, that's unfortunate, since there are a number of behavioral hints that could lessen their burden if they could find a physician prepared to offer wise counsel.[24] Many have been offered, even chosen from an assortment of pharmaceuticals and surgical procedures.[25] All the pharmaceutical and surgical options have marginal benefit-risk ratios at all ages — except for the frail elderly, for whom the ratio is prohibitive, and therefore these interventions are contraindicated. Frail elderly women feel no less embarrassed and stigmatized but are far more challenged physically, and often emotionally, to deal with incontinence. They deserve empathic advice regarding accessibility and frequency of toileting. Attention should be given to the timing and potency of diuretic therapy. And assistance may be needed in transferring to toilettes and in using incontinence garb correctly.

COGNITIVE IMPAIRMENT AND FRAILTY

The majority of frail elderly persons enjoy considerable cognitive competence. They may not be quite as sharp as they once were, but this could reflect a lack of reinforcement; for example, differential equations can challenge a distinguished mathematician who has not worked professionally for decades. Some elderly persons are forgetful, though many who are forgetful were always a bit absentminded. Some have acquired more forgetfulness than that. Some have acquired difficulties processing and recalling new information. This is termed minimal cognitive impairment. Some have acquired a severe and global cognitive deficit. This is termed dementia. Dementia has many causes, including Alzheimer's disease, which we have learned can afflict the elderly and is not just a "presenile" dementia, as was taught several decades ago. As was the case for depression, many medicines and a number of treatable medical conditions can cause dementia; the former should have been thwarted at the outset and the latter treated proactively. Furthermore, since there is no effective pharmaceutical treatment to prevent progression to dementia or reverse its manifestations, therapy is a combination of supportive care for the patient and the caregivers. Much has been written about this; my favorite reference for the general audience was written by P. Murali Doraiswamy and his colleagues.[26] However, there are advances in sorting out the continuum from forgetfulness to dementia, advances in understanding the biology of dementia, and lots of new pharmaceutical avenues actively being explored. All this is trumpeted in the media, often doing little justice to the state of the science.

The current criteria for diagnosing Alzheimer's, which have served as well as possible for twenty-six years, are based entirely on the patient's narrative. The diagnostic label is applied when there is no better explanation for a severe and global compromise in cognition that developed insidiously. The diagnosis of Alzheimer's when it is full blown is not a challenge. The challenge is in making the diagnosis when it is less obvious, when it is but "Possible" or "Probable." These categories are defined in the old criteria by considering the degree to which elements of cognition are compromised on various standardized psychometric tests. The application of these qualified diagnostic labels provokes as much anxiety in the clinician as it does angst in the patient and foreboding in the patient's intimate community. Maybe the fact that grandpa occasionally forgets his address or his neighbor's name is all there is to it; "grandpa's losing it," a touch of "senility." That would call for a supportive community and not the specter of a slide to a dreadful fate denoted by Alzheimer's.

Since the original criteria for Alzheimer's were formulated, there has been much scientific progress in the study of the full-blown disease. Changes in brain chemistry have been defined, some of which are apparent with modern imaging techniques, variations on MRI and PET scanning in particular. There are even chemicals that appear in the blood and spinal fluid that are associated with the process. All of these are lumped together under the rubric "biomarkers." The science of biomarkers continues apace in the hope that they relate to the cause of Alzheimer's and therefore to new therapeutic avenues. Already, there are randomized controlled trials of agents designed to interfere with the chemistry of particular biomarkers.

Could these biomarkers relate to prognosis? If so, they could be used to solve the riddle of early diagnosis, distinguishing forgetfulness from "Possible" or "Probable" Alzheimer's. This is a reasonable scientific question. From a clinical perspective, it is less pressing a question, since there is no therapy for early disease that will retard progression. In the clinical arena, the corollary question arises: "Am I better off for knowing?" But the scientific question caused the National Institute of Aging and the Alzheimer's Association to sponsor three working groups of prominent clinical and basic scientists with relevant expertise. Their consensus is that there is value in the measurement of biomarkers to predict which individuals with cognitive symptoms are likely to develop Alzheimer's. They have even proposed a category of preclinical Alzheimer's in which the patient has minimal if any cognitive impairment yet has one or more of the biomarkers. Implicit in such a category is the hypothesis that the biomarkers are not surrogate markers and therefore can be present in the absence of the disease but are directly involved in the progression to dementia. The analogy would be that a positive test for HIV means one will almost certainly progress to AIDS. However, for the Alzheimer's biomarkers, such an assertion is nothing more than a hypothesis, a rather tenuous hypothesis at that. Furthermore, if it is wrong, it will be quite harmful. The price of a "false positive" result is paid by the patient and the patient's family, whose fate was sealed, and by society in underwriting these tests, which are all expensive and some potentially harmful. The following study is an object lesson in why using biomarkers is likely to harm more than it helps.

The study was published by the Alzheimer's Disease Cooperative Study Group.[27] The major results are presented in Table 7. Nearly 800 septuagenarians with mild cognitive impairment volunteered. All had complained of insidiously progressive cognitive impairment, but none qualified even for "Possible" Alzheimer's by the old criteria. Three years later, 28 percent qualified for "Possible" or "Probable," but none had definite Alzheimer's. APOE ε4 is one of the better studied biomarkers; it is a genetic marker for predisposition to Alzheimer's.[28] It was present in about half of the volunteers. It was present in 163 (77 percent) of the 212 who progressed and in 260 (47 percent) of those who did not progress. This difference is scientifically meaningful because it is highly unlikely to have occurred by chance alone, but it is not clinically useful. This biomarker is present in too many who didn't progress and absent in too many who did to justify using it for prognosis and therefore for labeling or reassuring patients.

That begs the question of what we would do differently if we could identify early Alzheimer's patients. The study discussed above was actually a drug trial comparing the likelihood of progression if these volunteers were treated with vitamin E, donepezil (Aricept), or a placebo. There was no difference.

TABLE 7

Influence of APOE Ɛ4 on the Likelihood of
Progression from Minimal Cognitive Impairment to
"Possible" or "Probable" Alzheimer's Disease in the
Alzheimer's Disease Cooperative Study Group Trial

Volunteers	Number	Number That Progressed (%)
Total	769	212 (28)
APOE Ɛ4 carrier	426	161 (38)
APOE Ɛ4 absent	345	51 (15)

As I've made clear, no one should have a screening or a diagnostic test unless the test is accurate, the result is clinically meaningful, and something important can be done as a consequence to improve the patient's outcome. "Biomarkers" for Alzheimer's fail, many by all three standards. Biomarkers may be ready for prime time in terms of learning about etiology and even learning about prognosis, but not for labeling patients in the clinic. We have an obligation to discuss options for coping and to assure the safety of patients with mild cognitive impairment, but we cannot use biomarkers to justify more than that, certainly not to hang the curse of Alzheimer's disease on the patient or the patient's family.[29]

Mild cognitive impairment itself can lead to frailty and carries its own hazard for early death.[30] As is the case for physical disabilities, there is a reasonably consistent literature showing that programs of physical activity, including leisure activities, provide a stabilization of cognition if not a suggestion of improvement.[31] It has not been established whether this relates to the physical content of the exercise program or the personal interactions entailed in its execution. I suspect it requires both to see the benefit. I also suspect that socioeconomic status is playing a role, as leisure activities and exercise programs are more available to the wealthier segments of society, the segments with greater longevity and later onset of frailty.

Less clear is whether anything else matters. The conclusion of a "State-of-the-Science Conference" at the National Institutes of Health was not encouraging. A cadre of scientists with no particular axe to grind or overt conflicts of interest reviewed the world's scientific literature and concluded: "Few potentially beneficial factors were identified from the evidence on risk or protective factors associated with cognitive decline, but the overall quality of the evidence was low."[32]

That flies in the face of much marketing and common beliefs. For example, there is an industry based on the belief that dietary pattern matters. The data for benefit is not impressive and not consistent. For example, adherence to a Mediterranean diet affords no measurable benefit in France but a measurable benefit in New York City.[33] I am comfortable with the conclusion of the panel recently convened by the National Institutes of Health that there is no "solid evidence" that anything will prevent progressive cognitive decline.[34] And don't waste your money on Ginkgo biloba.[35]

Frail and Feeble

Exercise programs, social support, appropriate accommodations, medical counsel, and supportive social environment are often easier said than done. That was particularly true in post–World War II America, where mobility, diffusion of the community, and dispersion of the family became commonplace. Squalor and a lonely death was the fate of frail elderly persons who were less advantaged. This was a reproach to the community ethic that led to the Kerr-Mills Act in 1960, one of the last federal patches in the quilt of medical services for needy elderly people prior to the enactment of Medicare. Under Kerr-Mills, states could negotiate federal reimbursement for indigent care, particularly for the costs of institutionalizing indigent elderly people. For hospitals, this represented breathing room; for the nascent proprietary nursing-home industry, it was a boom that primed for the growth that was fueled by Medicare. In her treatise *In Sickness and in Wealth*, Rosemary Stevens uses Senator John Williams's pronouncement in Congress to illustrate the influence of profit seeking on this aspect of health care in America in 1969.[36]

> Since Medicare started there has been a remarkable increase in the number of chains entering the for-profit hospital and nursing home field. These groups, whose stocks have soared to unbelievable price-earnings ratios, are obviously lured by Medicare's generous reimbursement. . . . The fact that Medicare will pick up all of the costs of a 100 bed facility even if its total patient load consists of just five Medicare beneficiaries, the fact that there is no effective review of the utilization of beds and services in these facili-

ties, and the fact that the nursing home or hospital can choose the Government agent who will determine how much it is to be paid have certainly encouraged the get-rich-quick operations.[37]

Since the mid-1970s, the number of long-term-care beds has exceeded the number of acute hospital beds. Today, there are over 17,000 facilities approved under Medicare or Medicaid for the chronic institutionalization of elderly people. Most are proprietary, and all are to adhere to regulatory standards. This enterprise has captured the attention of myriad scholars, advocates, politicians, financiers, economists, regulators, geriatricians, and more — but few philosophers and even fewer poets. And it has molded the American social construction of frailty. Frailty has become synonymous with assisted living if not impending nursing-home care.

The notion of a facility dedicated to the compassionate shepherding of persons through the final transitions of life after completion of productive, interactive living made some sense when Kerr-Mills was formulated. In the mid-twentieth century, the temporal gap between "retirement" and death was narrow enough to support such a view. Over the past fifty years, the definition of "retirement" has changed and the gap has widened dramatically. Most of us will contend with years, even decades, of concern for the generation that preceded us and for the growing numbers of our birth cohort who are challenged to maintain peerage. "Nursing home" looms as an absorptive state, not as an empathic transition to the process of dying. We enter these "facilities" because we should and leave our intimates to cope with a mixture of relief, guilt, and foreboding. As a society, we have come to fear dependency and its attendant specter of nursing-home placement more than death. We fear being a burden and being without resources more than we fear loss of participation in the world we made. We have built and populated walled communities designed to succor us as the end of life approaches.

That is not to say that contemporary society has not attempted to revolt against the specter of the nursing home. The response is to build an assortment of way stations, all predicated on the principle that both quality and efficiency are best served if the patient is brought to where services are provided. No doubt this is true for services that demand expensive technology that can be shared. But does this tenet hold in any other instance? For the care of elderly people, the tenet lives under the rubric: "Continuum of Long-term Care." The intent is to provide continuity of care for any elderly person who dips a dependent toe into the mélange by orchestrating numerous interrelated services underwritten by multiple agencies. A Continuum of Long-term Care acknowledges the great variability in need. But it places the responsibility on the individual, the family, and the geriatric "providers"[38] to find the necessary services. The process fosters dependency. The compartmentalized menu of options, each with well-defended turf boundaries, causes elderly people to bump along its continuum from home to assisted living and eventually to the nursing-home terminus. Elderly people rarely fit perfectly within the providers' boundaries. They end up labeled—often to conform to the criteria of the provider rather than their own needs. Individuals change their living setting and location of care under psychological duress, if not distress.

The sterile definitions of services in the Continuum of Long-Term Care reduce the most personal aspects of independent living to service functions. No checklist does justice to the intimacies of toileting, bathing, sexuality, and eating. A narrow, literal approach to service delivery treats a bath or toileting as the goal without considering the manner and timing that shapes our very existence. All too often, autonomy is overridden, either by family members or by otherwise well-meaning professionals who need to serve expedience or their own proclivities rather than preserve intimacy and self-actualization.

The vortex of the Continuum of Long-Term Care leads to the dreaded nursing home. Its indelible image lies somewhere between a homeless shelter and a hospital: a smelly, run-down, unattractive warehouse filled with mentally and physically impoverished, half-dead people. "Nursing home" is the semiotic for "end-stage" and "hopeless." Care is very expensive (approaching $100,000 annually), and many families have to spend down to poverty levels to receive social support. Staff turnover in nursing homes is significant and in some cases over 100 percent per year.[39] The quality of care is often less than optimal, despite being highly regulated (only nuclear power plants have more regulations!).[40] Medical visits are often superficial and perfunctory. Moreover, whatever personal autonomy remained at admission is soon abandoned. There is little privacy, no choice in roommate, and no opportunity to lock the door. Inpatients must conform to institutional schedules of meals, rest, and recreation irrespective of past lifestyle choices. Personal, intimate care is often provided by minimally trained workers. Even high-end life-care communities minimize decisional control. It is a sad commentary that some elderly people would be better off committing a felony such as counterfeiting money:

in prison, their assets are preserved, their meals are guaranteed, and their health care is scrupulously monitored and fully covered.

For most people, particularly those who have been succored by their life course, the transitions from retirement to a ripe old age to frailty to dependency will play out over decades. The Continuum of Long-Term Care was in response to a different reality, a time when these transitions played out over mere years. It was designed to supplant or postpone nursing-home placement, as much because of the costliness of such placement as for the beneficence of avoiding it. It seemed reasonable to divorce this time of life from all that came before. It seemed reasonable to institutionalize the last chapter with a series of bricks-and-mortar way stations on the death march. It seemed expedient to populate the way stations with anonymous caregivers and wallpaper the way stations with reams of regulations.

As I explained in the preface, I have a familiarity with American nursing homes that dates back to my childhood. As a physician in training, I gained the experiences to qualify for board certification as a geriatrician. I have trained others to take that path, including Mark Williams, who worked with me on the study of dexterity in elderly women discussed above and who went on to a distinguished career as professor of geriatrics at the University of Virginia. Mark and I committed our careers as geriatricians to taking the stings out of the experience of aging in our society in a paper we wrote in 1983.[41] Health policy regarding frail elderly persons has gone terribly awry. The Continuum of Long-Term Care in America and the continuum of aging in America have grown dissonant. Aging is not a disease, and frail elderly persons are not a burden. Aging is a privilege of life in a resource-advantaged society, and the elderly, including frail elderly persons, enrich that society. Aging is a time of life that is as integral to our personal evolution as any other. And the aged are integral to the complexion of the community and to social cohesiveness, just as they were before they were advantaged by life experiences. Marginalizing this time of life deprives our communities of this lifeblood and denies the aged the sense of vitality that is the privilege of longevity. To marginalize elderly people today is to seal our own fate. Older people must be treated as people with a future and not only a past. Social policy must come to reflect this human value.

Until very recently, most people died at home. The fact of death could be certified on a slip of paper, but the process of dying recruited the most human of interactions. Family and community participated: visits, advice to the survivors, religious support, mourning rituals, farewells and blessings. It was a final affirmation of the person and his or her place in society. Today, most people die in institutions—in hospitals or nursing homes. Their care often is considered more a technical matter than one of moral concern. Too often in these institutions, there is more attention paid to the diseases than to persons, more scientific curiosity about the machinery of the body than consideration of the human values that make a life worthwhile, and too much focus on subspecialty technicalities and analgesic adjustments with no one looking at the needs of the whole person. Modern medical care has rendered the last illness fiscally burdensome, regardless of age. Modern society has rendered the last illness bereft of grace. Dying in a hospital, subjected to multiple traumatic, high-tech procedures and covered with tubes, has become a new symbol of contemporary death, today's *Danse Macabre*. Vain hopefulness supplants the touching comfort of goodbye. Dying has become aloneness.

The frail elderly deserve better, and we have enough science to inform the options. There is no need for yet another government program populated by strangers and designed in the abstract. There is a need to mobilize new community initiatives. "Naturally Occurring Retirement Communities" (NORCS) provide a model that could be transported into other settings. NORCS are communities in which the population has been stable for decades, so that the residents are aging together. Usually this means individuals are aging in parallel. There have been attempts to foster connections among the residents within such communities, so that medical care and community resources become integral to their daily lives rather than resources in times of crisis. Fredda Vladeck and Rebecca Segel of the United Hospital Fund in New York City are leaders in this approach. They have been studying a number of urban NORCS comprised of people who have aged in place.[42] My vision of a NORC differs; it should not mean a cohort aging together in a community but an integrated community that promotes awareness of neighbors and relationships across generations. Requisite resources and monies are sequestered behind the walls of the existing institutions and are now supplemented by the Community Living Assistance Services and Supports provisions of the Patient Protection and Affordable Care Act (H.R. 3590 and 4872). Let's supplant intergenerational communities in which the aging live side-by-side with those in which younger residents can benefit from the presence and experience of the elderly over time—knowing them and living with them and sharing life's challenges with them. And when it is the elderly's time to die, it should be in their own bed, in their own neighborhood, with the full acknowledgement of their extended community. Theirs should be communal memories. That is the higher calling.

7

THE REAPER

Most readers who arrived at adulthood in the 1960s recall family members and friends of the family who had died before age sixty. Usually a heart attack was a widow maker. These same readers who are now past sixty have seen few of their birth cohort struck down in this fashion. Yes, there have been tragedies, but no one takes such tragedies as facts of life any longer. This chapter takes the fact of our good fortune as a given and probes the implications for informed medical decision making at the end of life. If you arrived at adulthood in the 1960s, you will likely die an octogenarian, not a nonagenarian (see Figure 1 in chapter 1). Your time of death is predictable in terms of the decade. But it is not predictable in terms of the year—let alone the month, day, or hour.

- To plan to live beyond your ninth decade is unrealistic. For those whose life course has been colored by personal or fiscal deprivation, living into the ninth decade is a stretch.
- In your ninth decade, it doesn't matter how many diseases are vying to be the reaper or which disease ultimately wins out.
- In your ninth decade, both the quality of living and the quality of dying are primary health concerns.
- Everyone who is sixty already has significant atherosclerosis. By seventy it is impressive.
- Most who are sixty are harboring cancer, and nearly all who are seventy are harboring cancer.
- Nearly all who die in their ninth decade do so *with* many potentially lethal diseases, not *from* most of those diseases.

- It makes no sense to cure the diseases one will die *with* in the ninth decade and little sense to cure the disease that one will die *from* in the ninth decade if another is to take its place in short order.

All of these tenets have face value; they are obvious once stated. They are the reality that tests our quest to live beyond a ripe old age of eighty-five or so. It is a reality that seldom rests easily with an octogenarian who feels well. Rather, it is a reality that creates cognitive dissonance until death is at the door. It is no less difficult for others who are standing by and trying to make sense of the inevitability of death for another person.

Many of the insights I offer up in this book are gifts from patients who allowed me to share in their life experiences. A number of years ago, I had a patient who was a business executive who had retired to North Carolina. Sadly, his Golden Years were co-opted by a very rare disease that damaged the passages to the lung in bouts of inflammation that recurred unpredictably but diabolically frequently. I had no way to "cure" this disease or reliably prevent the recurrences. I could intervene during flares with steroids and supportive care, plus antibiotics when infection complicated the flares, as it often did. With each relapse, he lost ground; his course was slowly but inexorably downhill. What I haven't told you is that this gentleman was a long-term and very active member of the Hemlock Society, an organization that advocates for "dignified death" and for legalizing physician assistance in dying. At many levels, it was a privilege to know this man and his family.

His rocky course went on for years, rendering him more and more frail. The robust man with the vigorous lifestyle became a dim memory. Nonetheless, he enjoyed tight bonds with a very supportive family and was even capable of traveling some distance to participate in his daughter's wedding. We entered into a phase where I asked him at each flare whether he wanted to be admitted to the hospital, usually to an intensive-care unit for another valiant attempt at supporting him through the onslaught in the hopes that his disease would calm down again. This elegant man, this member of the Hemlock Society who had contemplated the process of dying in the abstract for decades, never told me it was time for less aggressive interventions. He never asked for more attention to comfort in an environment less harsh than an intensive-care unit. He died by millimeters, never willing or able to say "enough is enough." Between admissions, he became homebound, then chairbound but still able to read and enjoy the company of friends and family. He was willing to pay the price of progressively futile and unpleasant medical desperation to be able to see and know those he loved for *as long as possible*.

I do not dare project; I know not how I would feel and think if I had the option of postponing the time I would die. I know that such an option is never entirely mine to define. In the course of my career, I have been invited to teach and practice for lengthy intervals in other countries: a couple of years in Britain, semesters in France and Japan, and nearly as long in Israel and the antipodes. Unlike the usual fleeting visiting professorships, of which I've done many, these were intervals where I unpacked and was invited into the daily life of a medical community—one that was always highly sophisticated, both intellectually and technically.

My patient's life story would have played out quite differently in all of them. The diagnosis and the approach to management early in his course would have been similar. But as he became frail, inexorably so, it would be assumed by all that he was no longer a candidate for the relatively sparse intensive-care beds supported in other countries. This is not a withholding of care, or rationing, or any such thinking. It relates to the most rational use of finite resources. He would have been admitted to the hospital and treated aggressively in an ordinary hospital bed and not afforded the intubation and respirators we needed to support him through most of his last intensive-care admissions. He would have lived *as long as possible* in a different context of "possible." No other advanced country invests in as high a percentage of intensive-care-unit beds as the United States. Then again, no other country thinks marble lobbies and debt obligations are a sensible way to build a hospital. (I used to teach that the poorest countries minted the prettiest stamps. That's no longer true.) What's important to realize is that my patient's passing would have been sooner if he had been in another country, but it would have been similar from the perspective of his need to hang on to what he valued *as long as possible*.

Each culture defines "possible" according to its own community ethic. As David Reuben has written: "What is actually done for patients is driven by clinicians and patients and is determined by availability of services, access to these services, insurance, practice patterns, and patient and clinician choices."[1] America needs to understand this, and discuss this, and come to grips with it. My patient had insurance and access to a practice style that discourages any thoughts of "enough is enough." My patient's exposure to the Hemlock Society and my personal perspectives were overwhelmed by the American academic practice style. He was offered the option of attempting, at all cost, to postpone the inevitability of his death. In our setting and most others in America, the choice to not fight to the end — even to a bitter end — is considered un-American. This mindset fosters an enormous transfer of wealth in the exercise of turning the end bitter.

The particular saga that my patient lived out is not typical for dying in America or elsewhere. But I'm not so sure that his values and decisions are unique. "Meaningful life" and "quality in living" are anything but absolutes. I suspect that from my patient's perspective when he was in his prime and from the perspective of many members of the Hemlock Society, his fate in his last year would have been characterized as anything but "meaningful" or "quality." I suspect that from the vantage point of the well, his fate is a horrifying specter. But he was far from his prime. His point of reference was frailty, and from the perspective of the frail, there were redeeming features that were sufficient for him to persevere as long as possible. And he held on to life to the full extent that is underwritten by contemporary American society. I suspect that the desire to hold on to life is universal; our differences reflect our particular social and sociopolitical settings.

Guy de Maupassant (1850–93) captured this dynamic in his elegant short story *An Old Man*. Monsieur Daron is an octogenarian who cannot come to grips with his own mortality. He asks the doctor why another old man had died, and the doctor tells him, "He died because he died, that's all." Believing there must be a reason for death, he asks the man's age and learns that he had been eighty-nine. Monsieur Daron is relieved by this, concluding that "whatever it was, it wasn't old age" that killed him. I suspect very few octogenarians can do better than lip service to the inevitability of their own death. It's too abstract, even for those of us who have signed many a death certificate.

That does not mean that we are spared the need to confront the nitty-gritty of mortality, or that avoidance of the realities attendant on the process of dying is anything but foolhardy.

Advance Care Planning

Every octogenarian should have long before executed their last will and testament. Every octogenarian should have long before contingently authorized someone to make health-care decisions on their behalf should destiny deprive them of the competence to do so. In that event, the authorized individual would hold their health-care power of attorney. These are important legalities with ramifications that can be explained by many of the agents involved in their execution. Some of the ramifications are straightforward; there is nothing straightforward about defining the degree of incompetence at which you wish to relinquish control of health-care decisions. Global loss of competence, as in a vegetative state or coma from catastrophic brain damage, is an obvious reason for the designated surrogate to take over. Lesser degrees of cognitive impairment are more challenging, particularly if there is an element of reversibility, as may be the case with conditions that wax and wane or respond to therapy—including the "therapy" of eliminating drug toxicities.

It is difficult for anyone to foresee themselves dead, but thanks to media coverage and a more general exposure to cognitively impaired elderly individuals, it is less difficult to imagine becoming less competent. Discussing contingencies with the designated surrogate is as essential as the choosing of the surrogate. How else can this person know your preferences? These discussions are likely to be more productive in the presence of your health-care provider, particularly one who knows you well. They need to be frank and open, which requires trustworthiness on the part of all parties. And they need to be discussions that mature over time, reflecting both the state of your health and the state of your perspective on "life worth living." To this end, potential caregivers and surrogates should be included in interactions with physicians and other providers early in the process.[2]

There need to be frank discussions of your desires as to end-of-life care. Such desires can be codified, even detailed, in the formulation of advance directives. The need for advance directives does not pertain solely to acute illnesses or dementia but to all chronic diseases. It is not unusual for cognitive impairment to accompany severe organ-system malfunction, such as in end-stage cardiac or liver disease. Illness of this magnitude erodes self-awareness. The surrogate must be trusted to commandeer the decision-making process even if you do not think it is time for that. There is little that is formulaic about advance care planning. The discussions reflect all the humanity that the discussers bring to the challenge. We do know that these discussions improve the end-of-life experience for all involved. End-of-life wishes are more likely to be followed, and family members are likely to suffer less stress, anxiety, and depression.[3]

Discussions about advance care planning generally commence in response to high degrees of frailty or the specter of the terminal stages of acute or chronic diseases, often when the patient is already seriously if not critically ill. Such advance directives respond to the imminence of death by capitulation: "do not resuscitate," "pull the plug," "comfort care," and the like. This serves both the patient and the process of formulating an advance directive very poorly. Advance directives can serve much more than the last breath. They should be a rite of passage in this phase of life, living documents that reflect the life process rather than the preamble of the death certificate. Advance directives are natural to this last phase of life, just as contributing to a pension fund or purchasing life insurance marked earlier phases of life. Life insurance and tax-deferred annuities are more comfortable undertakings since one is underwriting something that is in the distant future, is somewhat abstract (in that it is hard to imagine the circumstance in detail), and is "good" because you are providing for yourself and your family in the future.

Discussions of advance directives when one is well are never so comfortable. They are always confounded by the sacrosanct heights that "hope" has attained through the twentieth and early twenty-first centuries. Like Monsieur Daron, we find it hard to accept that there may be no modern medical miracle to postpone our appointment with the Reaper. What do you mean by "nothing can be done for you that matters"? We shy away from dire prognostication because a declaration of hopelessness is considered inhumane, if not cruel.

Japanese medicine took this to heights that I couldn't imagine until I spent a semester teaching clinical medicine in the municipal hospital in Maizuru, a small city in Kyoto prefecture.[4] We had many patients with terminal cancer in beds in the open wards, each with intravenous lines dripping various medicines. Many had survived surgical interventions, all were wasting away, and all were surrounded by family members who assisted the staff with their nursing care. The "standard of care" dictated not only avoidance of discussions of prognosis; these patients and their families were also not to be told the diagnosis. All sorts of hopeful euphemisms colored bedside discussions. My students were a dozen highly selected resident physicians from the leading Japanese medical schools. We spent most of our time together discussing all manner of clinical content, including these patients. I asked them what they thought was going through the minds of these patients and their families. Did they imagine that none realized they had terminal disease, terminal cancer in particular? All, both doctors and patients, had access to Western media and to movies that focus on death and dying. The doctors did not deprive their patients of pharmaceutical care. How could they justify depriving them of the comfort of openness in saying and feeling their good-bye?

Japanese medicine has moved in the direction of openness since my teaching stint, though not as far as Western medicine has. Yet Western medicine still approaches prognosis in the terminal setting with discomfort, hesitancy, and distancing. Health-care surrogates, when questioned,[5] do not find this acceptable. They do not argue for assertions of hopelessness but rather for timely discussions about prognosis to help families begin to prepare emotionally and existentially, let alone practically, for the death of their loved one.

End-of-Life Care

The role of, if not the mandate for, advance care planning for the frail and the terminally ill is obvious. But the need for advance care planning reaches much farther back into the illness experiences of the aging population. This is feasible now that there is a robust science that defines prognosis. Medical decisions are contingent on the degree to which any treatment improves prognosis and the value one places on that improvement before embarking on any path. In contemporary America, the "value" denotes a personal assessment of the benefit/risk ratio; "value" is not a monetary metric. Neither "common practice" nor any war cry, such as "fight to the end," should be allowed to commandeer such informed, considered, and rational medical decision making. Let me illustrate this with two cases, both very close to home.

John Parker was a world-renowned hematologist. He was a legendary clinician and brilliant laboratory scientist who had mentored many a protégé, including one who was to go on to garner a Nobel Prize. He qualified as a prototypical aged worker. He was also a competent musician and serious jogger who had avoided all health-adverse behaviors, including tobacco abuse. One day, he noted lumps at the base of his neck, lumps that had the consistency of cancer. He ordered a chest X-ray on himself, only to learn that his lungs were riddled with abnormal tissue masses. We talked. I insisted that he have a biopsy; even though everything pointed to inoperable lung cancer, I felt strongly that we needed to exclude some unlikely but treatable possibilities. We did. He and I were well aware of the science that informed his options at this juncture. The best he could hope for from chemotherapy was a "response" to the drugs, but the response likely meant that he would die at the same time with a slightly smaller tumor mass. Yes, there were a few outliers in the trials, patients who lived many months longer than most, but he was not seduced by the lottery mentality; he knew his chances of being an outlier were nearly the same if he refused chemotherapy.

He discussed all this with his wife and family and opted to live with his lung cancer. He would forego all treatments designed to do violence to his cancer in the hopes of prolonging his life. He held his ground as word of his illness made its way into the oncology brotherhood, eliciting offers of experimental drugs that were in study protocols and some that were not even that far along. He was going to live as fully as he could for as long as he could. He published papers explaining his reasoning and perspective in the Groton School Quarterly (he was a Groton alumnus) and the North Carolina Medical Society Bulletin.[6] He put his estate in order and he returned to his laboratory to pursue his science with his customary passion and elegance.

The cancer cost him the ability to jog but took little else away for about six months. The next six months were inexorably downhill. He required opiates for pain relief and became ever more confined to his home. There were trips to the emergency room for pain control when a bone would fracture. There was hospice support and support from physicians who could understand what he was doing with this phase of his life. He died at home and is sorely missed to this day by many.

David was a psychotherapist who retired with his wife to Chapel Hill. He loved people and he loved life, and he pursued both a decade into retirement. He prided himself in his ability to put people at such ease that they turned to him for support with their personal problems, support that he provided simply as a willing friend. He also prided himself in his physique and athleticism. Aside from a cataract extraction, he had managed to find little reason to afford himself medical care throughout his life. This included foregoing an endoscopic screening examination for colorectal cancer. He knew my feelings about the rationale for such, as he had devoured every word of The Last Well Person when it was published in 2004. As we discussed in chapter 3, a single sigmoidoscopy is a defensible public-health recommendation.[7] A single sigmoidoscopy would have spared David the death he was to suffer.

In 2008 David started to bleed from his rectum. That got him his endoscopy and the diagnosis of rectal carcinoma. An MRI documented that the tumor extended into the wall of the bowel and that there were multiple tiny metastases in his liver. Cure was not possible. Removal of the tumor was advised as the best method for stopping the bleeding, which had become very confining and intolerable. However, it was possible, even likely, that he would require a colectomy because the tumor involved the rectal sphincters. I argued with David that this was a sensible palliative procedure that would greatly improve his quality of life during the early course of this terminal illness. For David, life with a colostomy and a pouch to collect stool was simply an intolerable specter. There was no arguing with him. The UNC oncologists offered an intervention that combined chemotherapy with radiation therapy. David examined the data documenting the limited effectiveness of all chemotherapeutic regimens that had been studied. He would not subject himself to adverse effects for such a puny likelihood of a puny benefit. He told the oncologists as much and felt that their response was a mixture of anger and disdain. They discharged him from their clinic.

The fallback was the radiation oncologist, who felt that high-dose radiation to the primary tumor should stop the bleeding. David found this an appealing option because he viewed it as "noninvasive" and self-limited. He either did not or could not hear my forewarning as to the complications of radiotherapy, particularly given the high doses his radiation oncologist felt were indicated. David put up with the misery of the course of radiation treatments, even providing support for others in the waiting room. He put up with the misery of the radiation-induced colitis, which was debilitating and more confining than the rectal bleeding. He emerged with no further rectal bleeding and having decided that he would no longer focus on anything that medicine or surgery might offer to prolong his life. He wanted to live as best he could until he died.

He recruited a young, brilliant physician from his circle of friends, a prominent AIDS specialist, to orchestrate the pharmaceutical aspects of palliation. He recruited from hospice a man who could share this stage of his life willingly and thoughtfully. His wife and family knew his wishes and found comfort in the knowing. His home became a gathering place for friends of all ages who turned to him for his friendship and wisdom. There is no doubt that modern medicine could have prolonged his dying; there is every doubt as to whether modern medicine could have prolonged his living. He died in his sleep.

John Parker and David leave substantial legacies, including object lessons for us in the way they made their choices.

Enough Is Enough

John Parker was comfortable with his decision, but he was dreadfully uncomfortable with the response of his peers. He wrote: "My biggest fear is that I will lose control and become the victim of well-intentioned colleagues, who through feelings of genuine altruism and interest in my welfare, will subject me to life-prolonging therapies I don't want." His admonition to these well-intentioned colleagues was: "Don't just do something; stand there." To "stand there" at the bedside of a patient who is faced with death from cancer is anathema for oncologists. They view it as a throwback to earlier generations, when the only option was to "stand there" promulgating the balm of concern and the poultice of bonding.

Contemporary oncologists have more important things to do. They have a science that is elucidating the biology of cancers and a pharmacology that is designed with that science in mind. They revel in examples where intervening is dramatically lifesaving, as with testicular cancer and some lymphomas. They realize that these are exceptions; randomized controlled trials of myriad agents in populations suffering with myriad cancers have proved disappointing. But they are the Captains of Chemotherapy and convinced they can tailor therapy to the advantage of their particular patient. They can find a way to get a "response." Their zeal is infectious, sweeping up patient after patient in their battle in the "War on Cancer." Some oncologists know no boundaries to their zeal, offering combination after combination — and damn the adverse effects. Some are cautious. Nearly all are ensconced in the fortress of peer review. This is another example of the folly of peer review, which values process over outcome. Some oncologists mutter about all this, but generally under their breath. Some speak out. In a compelling essay, Sarah Elizabeth Harrington and Thomas Smith used the data on improved survival from chemotherapy for four common solid tumors once they have metastasized to illustrate the modern exercise in futility (Table 8).[8]

John Parker had metastatic non-small-cell carcinoma of the lung. Now you know why his decision was informed and rational, and why I stood by his bedside. David had metastatic colon cancer at diagnosis. After the radiation therapy, he had had a belly full of modern medicine. His oncologists were furious with him because he chose to forego the possibility of another year of life on chemotherapy. For David, he wanted to live with his disease in the company of those he loved without the intrusion of trips to the hospital and all that entailed. Oncologists are convinced that such a

TABLE 8
Average Improvement in Survival from Diagnosis of Metastatic Disease through Standard Chemotherapeutic Treatments

Cancer	Standard Chemotherapeutic Treatments	Average Improvement in Survival from Diagnosis of Metastatic Disease
Lung (Non-small-cell)	First-line	About 3 months
	Second-line	About 2 months
	Second- or third-line	About 2 months
	Third- or fourth-line	<2% respond at all
Breast	Any and all treatments	Average survival has improved but drugs cannot account for this based on randomized controlled trials
Colon	Any and all treatments	From 9 to 22 months with new drugs
Prostate	First-line	About 2 months
	Second-line	No improvement in survival

decision is an example of noncompliance with their life view. They don't understand that it was not their life to view. David made an informed medical decision. John Parker's network of caring oncologists also needed to learn that it was not their life to view.

Notice the proviso (Table 8) regarding the "advances" for metastatic breast cancer. Metastatic breast cancer is a notoriously unpredictable disease—notorious from the perspective of oncologists trying to discern drug benefits, but reassuring from the perspective of patients. The course can be rapidly progressive, long dormant, staccato, and all in between. We don't know why. But the variability in the natural history bedevils drug trials because of the possibility that more patients with favorable biology will be randomized to one treatment to account for a spuriously favorable outcome. And there is another reason that "improved average survival" should be viewed with a skeptical eye. That reason is called "stage migration." Thanks to modern imaging techniques, we now can detect metastatic disease earlier than ever before. So patients who would have been labeled nonmetastatic a decade ago are now labeled metastatic and entered into trials for treating metastatic disease. However, compared to the patients labeled metastatic a decade ago because of an obvious spread of the cancer, these new-age patients have earlier disease and would be expected to survive longer on that basis. So "stage migration" is the tendency to label early disease as late disease and be fooled by the improved survival. The upshot is the proviso in Table 8.

Don't get me wrong. There are metastatic cancers for which oncology has interventions that offer substantial benefits. I am not urging you to take a diagnosis of metastatic cancer as reason to avoid further discussions with an oncologist. Rather, I am trying to teach you and the person you choose as a surrogate how to participate in such discussions so that you are fully informed and can make decisions that truly reflect your desires. I am hopeful that some day we will see truly effective treatments for more metastatic cancers. But that day has yet to dawn for the commonest of cancers. And that fact has yet to dawn on the commonest of oncologists. As for the public, it's a dirty little secret. Furthermore, we stand a better chance of disabusing the public than of altering the behaviors of the oncology community. They hide in their peer review.

Take the recent Cabot Case Record of the Massachusetts General Hospital (MGH).[9] This is a century-old weekly exercise where a respected clinician is asked to discuss a particularly challenging case before the staff and trainees at the MGH. The transcript is published in the vaunted *New England Journal of Medicine* and provides a teaching instrument for legions of doctors around the world. Hyman Muss, currently my colleague at UNC, where he is director of geriatric oncology, discussed the case of an eighty-five-year-old woman with early breast cancer detected by mammography. Nothing about the case makes sense: the cancer was detected by "routine mammography," she underwent a lumpectomy, no metastases were found in her lymph nodes, she underwent radiation therapy, and some chemotherapy was thrown in as a bonus. If she was fifty-five years old, this sequence would hardly be defensible. At eighty-five, it is gross overtreatment—Type 2 Medical Malpractice, in my terminology—at every step of the way. To be charitable, Muss points out that much that was done was "controversial." But I'm not inclined to be charitable about this particular case; this is a case report of unconscionable overtreatment sanctioned by American medicine by virtue of this publication.

I am more willing to be charitable about the state of oncology at the MGH, perhaps because it is my internal medicine residency alma mater. A glimmer of reflection appears to be creeping into their approach to treating metastatic cancers. They are thinking about treating the patient as well as the cancer. John Parker died from metastatic non-small-cell lung cancer. He chose what would be termed "palliative care" to the exclusion of chemotherapy. The oncology world was put off by his choice fifteen years ago and would be so today. That explains the design of a randomized controlled trial for treating metastatic non-small-cell lung cancer at the MGH today.[10] They recruited 151 patients with newly diagnosed metastatic non-small-cell lung cancer into the trial. All would be afforded "standard oncologic care," which means whatever combinations of chemotherapy and radiotherapy the oncologists deemed appropriate and the patients acceded to. Half were also given "palliative care" from the get-go, which means frequent visits from trained personnel with attention to their fears, anxieties, symptoms, and other aspects of the quality of their lives. Over half of these 151 patients were dead within a year. Those who had "palliative care" experienced less depression, less anxiety, and generally a better quality of life. They also tended to refuse chemotherapy and aggressive end-of-life care more often. And they survived an average of nearly three months longer. The message about the utility of palliative care for metastatic cancer is not lost on anyone. But no one is wondering out loud whether the chemotherapy and radiotherapy added anything of substance to the palliative care.

There is more than the folly of peer review at work here. Oncologists are pawns in an industry dedicated to developing drugs and assaying their effectiveness. Oncology is big business. It is so big that the Research Triangle in North Carolina has seen fit to construct three separate "cancer centers," each costing over $250 million in private or, in the case of UNC, taxpayer monies. Each of these centers devotes much space and personnel to infusion beds and pharmaceutical trials. The former are necessary to administer the ever-growing list of "biologics," drugs that are molecules that cannot be administered by mouth and often require doses too great for any route of administration other than through the vein. Those agents that have been licensed by the FDA are generally underwritten by private medical insurance and Medicare, often to the tune of many tens of thousands of dollars per treatment. There are all sorts of financial arrangements that turn infusion clinics into cash cows for the cancer centers or for private oncologists, who nearly always have their own infusion clinics.

Don't for one moment think that Medicare, let alone the private medical-insurance industry, is bucking the trend to infuse exceedingly expensive agents into patients with metastatic disease despite minimal efficacy. Medicare is under great political pressure to provide the "very best," regardless of the cost (or of the fatuous nature of "best"). Any perception otherwise will elicit screams of rationing from all sorts of stakeholders, as well as from the desperate patients and their families who are encouraged to believe that treatments that are disappointingly marginal in efficacy in trials might save their lives. The same pressure is brought on the FDA at the licensing stage and post-marketing stage.

In the summer of 2010, the FDA received a letter from Nancy G. Brinker, leader of the Susan G. Komen for the Cure breast cancer treatment advocacy group, demanding that the agency maintain its approval of Genentech's Avastin for women with life-threatening metastatic breast cancer. "We recognize the benefits of Avastin overall are modest," wrote Ms. Brinker. "However, we do know that for some women, Avastin offers a greater than modest benefit." Avastin is a triumph of molecular biology, a biologic that in laboratory models can stop metastases from co-opting the blood supply of the normal tissue. Without a new blood supply, the cancer cannot live, let alone grow. Unfortunately, the randomized controlled trials demonstrated minimal if any benefit. Of course, some women treated with Avastin seemed to live longer, but then again some women treated with a placebo also lived longer. Ms. Brinker is leading the Komen advocates down the lottery mentality pathway, ignoring the power for rationality that is built into the design of randomized controlled trials. But Ms. Brinker wields a mighty powerful political bludgeon.

There is another perverse aspect to this dialectic. Almost everyone with health insurance in America is insured by their employer. For those of us on Medicare, the Medicare fund is our de facto employer. In theory, the cost of health insurance is lowered by such an arrangement because the employer is assuming the risk for unanticipated costs. All of these self-insured employers turn to the private health-insurance industry to process the claims. The health-insurance companies function as "cost plus" providers, meaning that they are compensated for their efforts by a negotiated percentage of the cash throughput. The more money spent on "health care," the greater the yield for the health-insurance industry, which translates into their obscene executive salaries and bonuses and perks. There is no financial motivation for the health-insurance industry to cut the cost of health care by arguing against marginal therapies or their costliness.

And don't be fooled into thinking that randomized controlled trials are designed solely with truth as the goal. Most of the trials are very large, complex, and costly because of the realization that the best to be hoped for is slightly more benefit than toxicity. Statistical theory holds that in a perfect world, with perfectly matched subjects and exquisitely accurate outcome measurements, one can reliably detect tiny effects by studying ever-greater numbers of subjects. The trials are costly, but not simply because of their size: oncologists and their institutions are the recipients of a good deal of compensation for participating. Most major medical centers are now competing with private "Contract Research Organizations" for the rewards of performing trials. "Cancer centers" are devoted to this profitable exercise. Many "trials" are actually "seed" trials, in which the object is more marketing through familiarity than seeking new information. The amount of money involved, coupled with the large and messy data sets, is a setup for biased analyses of data if not malfeasance. Such has become a blight on industry-sponsored trials, and not just in oncology.[11]

The upshot is that trials sponsored by industry are more likely to be published quickly if they are deemed positive and more likely to be deemed positive than trials of the same agents with nonindustrial sponsors. The realization of this bias has led to much wringing of hands and tweaking of the process. My response is that we should no longer undertake these enormous trials because tiny effects are clinically meaningless. We should be looking for clinically dramatic advances with targeted small trials, because data demonstrating large effects (or not) do not lend themselves to subliminal or intentional massaging and torturing in their analysis. And we should expunge all the conflicts of interest that sup off this largesse—and I mean expunge and not just decry. I mean more than fiscal penalties for immoral behaviors. I mean more than censorship. I want licensure put at risk contingent on the successful completion of remedial programs like the ones we promulgate for physicians impaired by substance abuse. And I want an open discussion of the fashion in which academic institutions, particularly medical schools, have partnered with external agencies. Annalee Yassi and her colleagues examined these relationships in detail and concluded: "In becoming servants of government or corporatism, universities have become less vital to society and are failing in their mission to promote social justice and sustainability. Strong measures are needed to restore public trust."[12] The twenty-first century demands new standards for ethical behavior that do not tolerate conflicts of interest that place patients at any disadvantage.

Before I end this diatribe, I need to emphasize that while oncology is a poster child for this scenario, it is not the only poster child. For example, we discussed interventional cardiology in detail in chapter 4. Patients older than seventy-five were excluded from nearly all trials of treating symptomatic coronary artery disease, although a glance at Medicare data demonstrates that this age group has not escaped the net of interventional cardiologists and cardiovascular surgeons. A decade ago, the investigators participating in the Trial of Invasive versus Medical Therapy in Elderly Patients (TIME) published the short-term results, arguing that the slight improvement in reports of symptoms was worth the excess mortality of the procedures. The results at one year are even less compelling.[13] It requires a committed cardiologist[14] to argue that anyone can identify any elderly patients for whom invasive therapy for symptomatic coronary artery disease makes sense. Furthermore, no patient or surrogate should agree to invasive therapy, such as biventricular pacing or bypass grafting for heart failure, without demanding to see and discuss the data that supports such a recommendation.

To give another example, there is no doubt that renal dialysis ranks among the greatest therapeutic advances of the twentieth century. It prolongs the life of patients with end-stage renal failure. But there is nothing simple about the process, nor does it substitute fully for the sense of well-being that is compromised by renal failure. In testimony to our national ethic, Medicare and Medicaid underwrite dialysis for any patient with end-stage renal disease who desires to prolong his or her life in this fashion. This is an enormously expensive undertaking that underwrites the many very profitable dialysis centers that dot the landscape, as well as other stakeholders. One particularly disconcerting stakeholder is the biotechnology firm Amgen. Patients on dialysis are anemic and generally feel weak. Amgen isolated the hormone erythropoietin, which drives the bone marrow to make more red blood cells. Early studies suggested a slight improvement in the sense of well-being of dialysis patients who are treated with erythropoietin. The cost of this treatment is now the same order of magnitude as the monies expended on nursing salaries at dialysis centers. The benefit derived from this treatment was never impressive. What has become clear, however, is the harmfulness of raising the blood counts: it increases the risk for serious cardiovascular events and death.[15] This does not mean that erythropoietin is no longer administered, only that it is administered in lower doses — and to an ever-growing number of patients placed on dialysis. In the past decades, the notion that no American should die of renal failure without being on dialysis has entered the nursing homes. More and more, frail elderly patients who develop end-stage renal disease are transported to dialysis centers for their weekly treatments. This may do wonders for their blood chemistries, but it is associated with a substantial decline in their functional status. The frail elderly would be better served by palliative care.[16]

Surviving Rescue Care

Many, many people are hospitalized with acute major illnesses only to emerge better, often no worse for wear. Trauma, abdominal catastrophes, infectious diseases, and so much more have yielded to the medical and surgical advances of the past fifty years. Many people are also hospitalized to manage acute complications or flares of their chronic diseases, often to good effect. Many used to be hospitalized in order to facilitate consultative input and thereby expedite a diagnostic evaluation. This latter contingency is unusual today, since it has been deemed a waste of resources by those who have never attempted to sort out a diagnostic enigma in an outpatient; America has deemed it preferable to burden such patients with multiple return trips for that purpose. In the distant past, the hospital was also used as a setting for the patient to collect him- or herself, come to grips with the ramifications of illness, seek supportive care, "rest," and the like. This caring function was defunded twenty years ago. I have spent a great deal of my life as a physician in UNC Hospitals caring for patients faced with circumstances such as these. Theirs are not the circumstances we are considering in this chapter.

We are considering the frail elderly and the elderly faced with terminal illnesses. We are exploring the circumstances in which reversibility is a very time-limited goal, if it is a reasonable goal at all. What is the role of hospitalization in such a circumstance? More broadly, what is the role of medical intervention in such a circumstance? There is no simple or single answer; there are too many variables to "such a circumstance." The people, their disease(s), their community support systems, and their medical support systems are anything but uniform. That truth may be a thorn in the side of health-policy wonks, but it is a truth that makes life interesting, that nurtures poets, and that is the calling to all who devote their lives to ministering to the ill. The prerequisites for providing optimal care of the frail elderly were discussed in the previous chapter and are summarized as follows:

- Physicians and others involved in the care of the frail elderly need extensive knowledge of the aging process.
- Physicians and others involved in the care of the frail elderly need extensive knowledge of the prognosis of any confounding or intercurrent diseases.
- Care must be proactive and provided with continuity across diverse settings and over the course of the aging process.
- Care by various caregivers must be closely coordinated.
- Caregivers, patients, and surrogates must interact and communicate effectively over time. Contingencies regarding intercurrent and confounding diseases must be established as early in their course as possible.
- Hospitals have a role that needs definition and demands enlightenment regarding the special needs of the frail elderly who are acutely ill.

All of this is possible if we shift the priorities of Medicare from the futile and useless to the needs of an aging society.[17] Furthermore, there is an urgent need for this shifting, a need that relates only partly to the neglected needs of the elderly. It relates to the fact that the current approach that offers up the option of acute hospitalization for acute intercurrent illness and acute decompensation is more lethal than it is salutary.

The frail elderly seldom escape acute care and critical-illness hospitalization unscathed. Those who have no demonstrable cognitive impairment when admitted are far more likely to develop dementia after discharge than similar frail elderly who did not suffer an acute hospitalization.[18] Frail or not at admission, the elderly run a considerable risk of never returning to their prehospitalization level of physical functioning.[19] Hospitalization is a difficult experience for everyone; it can be quite disorienting for older persons, particularly the frail elderly who can develop frank delirium. Management is challenging, as restraints and drugs to calm them down are all-too-often counterproductive. Much effort is expended in keeping the patient alert and oriented, usually by recruiting family as bedsitters. It turns out that delirium is a symptom of greater degrees of frailty. These patients do poorly after discharge, with considerable likelihood of dementia and mortality.[20]

Over 10 percent of patients, particularly elderly patients, recover from critical illnesses very slowly. In order to free up the expensive acute-care hospital beds, the Centers for Medicare and Medicaid Services is under-

TABLE 9

Disposition of Patients over Age Sixty-Five Who Were Admitted to Intensive Care Units in 2006

Patients	Number Admitted	Discharged Home (%)	Discharged to Skilled Nursing Facility (%)	Discharged to Long-Term Acute Care (%)	Died (%)
All	1,637,581	57.7	24.6	2.5	15.3
Ventilated	227,152	20.6	25.1	8.7	45.7

writing a new inpatient care model, the long-term acute-care hospital, to serve as a way station between the acute-care hospital and the skilled nursing facility or rehabilitation hospital. Long-term acute-care hospitals are growing like mushrooms, hospitalizing over 40,000 patients in 2006. They are testimony to a very limited view of health economics. In 2006 nearly 2 million patients over age sixty-five were admitted to intensive-care units.[21] The likelihood of discharge and patients' disposition if discharged are illustrated in Table 9. About 55 percent of elderly patients who require mechanical ventilation survive to leave the intensive-care unit, and half of them do well enough to return home — though nearly all are worse for wear, as we've discussed. The middle ground between death and home is a quagmire. About half who are sent to long-term acute hospitals are alive a year later. Those discharged to skilled nursing facilities fare better, but not that much better; a quarter will be dead in six months.[22] Hospitalized elderly patients who are not so critically ill as to require treatment in an intensive-care unit also have substantial three-year mortality but die at about a third the rate.

There are several inescapable conclusions. Only a minority of critically ill elderly patients are well served by intensive medical and surgical therapy. If they are so ill that they require mechanical ventilation, the exercise is futile at best for most.[23] And if they die and are successfully resuscitated, the yield in terms of discharge from the hospital, let alone functional return or even return home, is dismal.[24]

To Resuscitate, or Not to Resuscitate

Advance directives and end-of-life planning need to realize the limitations of rescue therapy. If thoughtful proactive medical interventions cannot forestall critical illness in the frail elderly, it is highly unlikely that aggressive interventions can bring one back from the precipice of critical illness. Some intensivists, such as Theodore Iwashyna of the University of Michigan,[25] argue that these realities are a rallying cry for improving the lot of the elderly who manage to become survivors of intensive-care unit admissions. For me, this is a priority, but not the top priority. A goodly percentage of these critically ill elderly succumb despite all the bells and whistles of the modern acute-care hospital. In fact, the more dramatic, invasive, or wretched the heroics, the less likely is survival. A goodly percentage of those who survive the hospitalization do not survive long after discharge, regardless of the disposition. And a goodly percentage who do survive as long as their peers who were not hospitalized survive with a severely compromised level of function and quality of life.

For me, the top priority is to identify those few elderly for whom hospitalization is likely to offer substantial benefit in the longer term and hospitalize them. All the others for whom the acute illness is but the last straw deserve a far kinder, caring, supportive fate. When an eighty-six-year-old woman is progressively feeble from congestive heart failure despite optimal medical therapies, what right do we have to offer her death during, or near to, or from acute hospitalization? What ethic is served when the underlying disease is irreversibly end-stage if we attempt to alter the proximate cause of death? She, her family, her surrogates, and her physicians are serving her best by allowing her to pass gently into the night. And if there are any concerns as to the gentleness with which this is to play out, there are individuals committed to calming the waters with professionalism and expertise. Some are to be found in the hospice movement, some in the clergy, and some in the larger caring community. No one needs to die alone, afraid, abandoned—but no one needs to die in an acute hospital unless there was good reason a priori. This is true if a fellow human being is dying of end-stage heart disease[26] or is fully demented.[27] When it is one's time, it is one's time. All societies have understood this in the past. It is only modern societies that are deluded by the myths of medical magic to think otherwise. This is part of life.

8

AUTUMN

I was walking on the beach hand-in-hand with Lucy, my larger-than-life six-year-old granddaughter. We were breathing in life at its finest and at its fullest. Out of the blue, Lucy looked up and said, "Peepa, I want to stay a kid because kids don't die." Leaving aside the sad truth that she's not 100 percent correct, for me this was a Kantian moment. Of course, I didn't say that to Lucy, but I hope I can live long enough to explain it to her. For now, we settled for a discussion of joyful moments together in the present.

There are two ways to conceptualize time. Both are familiar, but only one is generally recognized as "time," the empirical, Newtonian, reliable, predictable, linear scales that we need to mark events: seconds, minutes, years, and so on. In *Critique of Pure Reason*, Immanuel Kant (1724–1804) offered an alternative conception of time. Kant explores the fashion in which the mind imposes time on our experiences. Kant's treatment of this notion is as dense as any of his writings, but also as important. It speaks to such parlance as "time flies" or "time drags" or "time goes quickly when I'm having fun." Such parlance is sensible because we accept the interactive nature of experience and perception. And we generally accept it—except when it comes to advance care planning and end-of-life decisions. When death is inevitable and imminent, advance care planning and end-of-life discussions are tolerated by many, encouraged by some. But when the specter of death is based on prognosis, many patients prefer to take things one day at a time rather than contemplate serious illness and death.[1] In our culture, there is a "wide-spread and deeply held desire not to be dead."[2] It is so entrenched that dispassionate discussions of end-of-life decision making can elicit passionate reproaches about "death panels."[3] And it grows ever more entrenched as society is plied with the putatively lifesaving medical miracle of the month. Perhaps *Rethinking Aging* will arm elderly people with the desire for accurate scientific information and the wherewithal to listen actively to its exposition. But there is no way to expunge uncertainties about the future from the life course. Prognosis is a stochastic concept, a statement of the likelihood you will or will not do poorly in a finite period of time. It is possible to stratify older adults into categories that predict four-year mortality, but the categories are rather broadly constructed and rely heavily on the obvious, such as age and frailty.[4] The fact is that if you look at the year prior to death for community-dwelling older adults, the course of disability does not follow a predictable pattern.[5] Prognosis is not a knell; it's enlightenment.

I have written *Rethinking Aging* so that readers will learn to think of prognosis as a call for advance care planning even if that planning proves unnecessary. I want prognosis to signal a change in the parlance of time from "my time is limited" to "my time is valuable, too valuable not to capture every moment I can." Whether robust or frail, if you have the mental capacity to do so, then make time slow down. In that context, advance care planning is a part of staying alive and not of dying.

But we will die.

Why Do We Die?

We have a great deal of epidemiology speaking to the likely time of death.

We have a great deal of clinical information speaking to the proximate cause of death.

We have a rapidly advancing science as to the molecular biology of the death of our cells.

But as to why we die, we have but a plethora of theories. Many are metaphysical. I won't go there. But many are based on biological constructs that I find thought provoking. None is completely satisfying, most defy testing, and none is exclusive. They tend to cluster into several categories.

- The Cartesian image of our body as a machine that simply wears out is untenable unless coupled with the notion that the biology that maintains the machine wears out. Such a formulation allows for progressive limitation in the biological availability of the building blocks and imperfections in the maintenance procedures. Such a conceptualization resonates with the "Six Sigma" formulation that dominates the Western industrial establishment, a formulation that seeks efficiency and perfection in industrial processing. If we learned to do it right and always did it right, output and profitability would improve. The mathematical methodology and perspective was introduced into the Japanese automotive industry by W. Edwards Deming (1900–1993) a half century ago. Six Sigma was introduced by Bill Smith into Motorola twenty-five years ago. It is a perspective that treats the workforce as part of a machine to be well greased. It may work for building Toyotas, but the recent attempt to introduce it into patient care is dying because the "process," caring for the patient, is anything but a robotic undertaking; and the "product," the well-being of a patient, is anything but unitary. The same factors limit any therapeutic approach to the "body is a machine to be maintained or it will die."

- The Darwinian theory as to why we die also must be contended with. Population genetics speaks to reproductive success, not longevity. There is no evolutionary pressure to develop biology to live beyond reproductive years. Longevity is a superfluous bonus. I have been fascinated with these notions since my early days as a geneticist working with fruit flies. This was long before fruit fly genetics became a focus for molecular biology. Early on, the biology of the entire fly was the focus, as in my work in behavior genetics. Others showed that if you delay reproduction in fruit flies, they live longer.[6] It's as if there is some biological pressure to maintain normal biology until the next generation is aboard. We have no idea how this happens.

- Finally, the biology of cell death offers up some interesting possibilities that offer molecular counterparts to the above. When cells divide normally, the DNA is reproduced in the progeny. But it turns out that with each division, the copying is programmed to be imperfect. The ends of the chromosomes are likely to be frayed and shortened over time. Clearly, there is an intrinsic biological clock at play. Maybe it's set for around eighty-five years of cells dividing. "Maintenance" becomes the notion of allowing this to play out. Of course, there are those who are convinced they can tie up the frayed ends of their DNA and live forever. These include the collaboration at the Rockefeller Institution a century ago between the Charles Lindbergh and Dr. Alexis Carrel, the Nobel Prize–winning pioneering surgeon.[7] Don't hold your breath.

We will die. And we will leave behind the mystery of our dying.

> *Everywhere ... the consciousness of the living still experiences a fearfulness before the mystery of death, a shuddering before its sacredness, and there is still something uncanny in the silence which accompanies the final parting of someone who was even just now among the living.*[8]

Into the Night

A great many of you who are reading this book will live to be octogenarians. Most of our forebears, most who died a generation or two back, never saw such a ripe old age. There have always been outliers, even very old people who considered themselves fortunate for their longevity. But they were outliers. We, a great many of us, are the recipients of the privilege of making something important, special, and pleasing of our lives through the seventh and even eighth decades. There is much we can do and more we can avoid to realize this promise of longevity. There is much we can do and more we can avoid while we are well and if we are frail. We can even do much to turn the process of dying into a valuable time of living that holds on to fulfillment rather than a time of thrashing. *Rethinking Aging* is designed to teach you how to recruit medicine to your goal of living life fully. But you will die.

There is a literature on the experience of dying generated by interviewing patients who recovered from cardiopulmonary resuscitation. I do not know what to make of these narratives. I am more drawn to poetry. We started the book with Shakespeare's seventy-third sonnet. We will end it with "To Autumn" by John Keats. Keats was born in 1795, the son of a stable attendant. In 1810 he apprenticed to an apothecary-surgeon, and in 1815 he entered the medical school of Guy's Hospital in London. A year later, he left Guy's to spend his life as a poet. At age twenty-three, he nursed his brother Tom through terminal tuberculosis. The following year, he realized that he, too, was infected. By twenty-five, he was quite ill from the disease, feverish, thin, and coughing up blood. That was 1820. He traveled to Italy, hoping that a gentler climate would be helpful. He died on February 23, 1821, at age twenty-six. But he lived a long life, a rich and full life, and he left a most extraordinary legacy of a way to look at and think about life and the world we live in, to find both the sensual and the beautiful.

Some of Keats's most powerful works emerged in his last years, when he was so ill. Because of his medical training and experience nursing Tom, Keats knew and understood his circumstance as a dying man. Most scholars point to his "La Belle Dame sans Merci" as an uplifting requiem in which Keats extols the delightful sensations of living. We are to savor life, the poet tells us, rather than dwell on the negative or tragic sides of our existence. This was one resilient young man. "To Autumn" was written in this spirit.

TO AUTUMN

1.

Season of mists and mellow fruitfulness,
    Close bosom-friend of the maturing sun;
Conspiring with him how to load and bless
    With fruit the vines that round the thatch-eves run;
To bend with apples the moss'd cottage-trees,
    And fill all fruit with ripeness to the core;
      To swell the gourd, and plump the hazel shells
With a sweet kernel; to set budding more,
    And still more, later flowers for the bees,
    Until they think warm days will never cease,
      For summer has o'er-brimm'd their clammy cells.

2.

Who hath not seen thee oft amid thy store?
    Sometimes whoever seeks abroad may find
Thee sitting careless on a granary floor,
    Thy hair soft-lifted by the winnowing wind;
Or on a half-reap'd furrow sound asleep,
    Drows'd with the fume of poppies, while thy hook
      Spares the next swath and all its twined flowers:
And sometimes like a gleaner thou dost keep
    Steady thy laden head across a brook;
    Or by a cyder-press, with patient look,
      Thou watchest the last oozings hours by hours.

3.

Where are the songs of spring? Ay, where are they?
    Think not of them, thou hast thy music too,—

While barred clouds bloom the soft-dying day,
    And touch the stubble-plains with rosy hue;
Then in a wailful choir the small gnats mourn
    Among the river sallows, borne aloft
        Or sinking as the light wind lives or dies;
And full-grown lambs loud bleat from hilly bourn;
    Hedge-crickets sing; and now with treble soft
    The red-breast whistles from a garden-croft;
        And gathering swallows twitter in the skies.

NOTES

ALL URLS ARE ACCURATE AS OF JANUARY 2011

Chapter 2

1. A. Bowling and P. Dieppe, What is successful ageing and who should define it?, *British Medical Journal* 2005; 331: 1548–51.

2. C. M. Callahan, C. A. McHorney, and C. D. Mulrow, Successful aging and the humility of perspective, *Annals of Internal Medicine* 2003; 139: 389–90.

3. B. H. Strand, E.-K. Grøholt, Ó. A. Steingrímsdóttir, T. Blakely, S. Graff-Iversen, and Ø. Næss, Educational inequalities in mortality over four decades in Norway: Prospective study of middle aged men and women followed for cause specific mortality, 1960–2000, *British Medical Journal* 2010; 340: c654, doi:10:1136/bmj.c654.

4. T. Chandola, J. Ferrie, A. Sacker, and M. Marmot, Social inequalities in self reported health in early old age: Follow-up of prospective cohort study, *British Medical Journal* 2007; doi:10.1136/bmj.39167.439792.55 (27 April).

5. J. P. Mackenbach, I. Stirbu, A.-J. R. Roskam, M. M. Schaap, G. Menvielle, M. Leinsalu, and A. E. Kunst for the European Union Working Group on Socioeconomic Inequalities in Health, Socioeconomic inequalities in health in 22 European countries, *New England Journal of Medicine* 2008; 358: 2468–81.

6. M. Minkler, E. Fuller-Thomson, and J. M. Guralnik, Gradient of disability across the socioeconomic spectrum in the United States, *New England Journal of Medicine* 2006; 355: 695–703.

7. K. Fiscella and D. Tancredi, Socioeconomic status and coronary heart disease risk prediction, *Journal of the American Medical Association* 2008; 300: 2666–68; L. Berkman and A. M. Epstein, Beyond health care — Socioeconomic status and health, *New England Journal of Medicine* 2008; 358: 2509–10; P. M. Lantz, J. S. House, R. P. Mero, and D. R. Williams, Stress, life events, and socioeconomic disparities in health: Results from the Americans' Changing Lives Study, *Journal of Health and Social Behavior* 2005; 46: 274–88.

8. S. T. Lindau and N. Gavrilova, Sex, health, and years of sexually active life gained due to good health: Evidence from two U.S. population based cross sectional surveys of ageing, *British Medical Journal* 2010; 340: c810, doi:10.1136/bmj.c810; P. M. Lantz, E. Golberstein, J. S. House, and J. Morenoff, Socioeconomic and behavioral risk factors for mortality in a national 19-year prospective study of U.S. adults, *Social Science and Medicine* 2010; 70: 1558–66.

9. P. A. Braveman, C. Cubbin, S. Egerter, K. S. Marchi, M. Metzler, and S. Posner, Socioeconomic status in health research: One size does not fit all, *Journal of the American Medical Association* 2005; 294: 2879–88.

10. D. M. Mirvis and D. E. Bloom, Population health and economic development in the United States, *Journal of the American Medical Association* 2008; 300: 93–95.

11. A. Bowling, Enhancing later life: How older people perceive active ageing, *Aging and Mental Health* 2008; 12: 293–301.

12. H. M. Orpana, J.-M. Berthelot, M. S. Kaplan, D. H. Feeny, B. McFarland, and N. A. Ross, BMI and mortality: Results from a national longitudinal study of Canadian adults, *Obesity* 2010; 18: 214–18, doi:10.1038/oby.2009.191.

13. L. Flicker, K. A. McCaul, G. J. Hankey, et al., Body mass index and survival in men and women aged 70 to 75, *Journal of the American Geriatrics Society* 2010; 58: 234–41.

14. Prospective Studies Collaboration, Body-mass index and cause-specific mortality in 900,000 adults: Collaborative analyses of 57 prospective studies, *Lancet* 2009; 373: 1083–96.

15. K. M. Flegal, B. I. Graubard, D. F. Williamson, and M. H. Gail, Cause-specific excess deaths associated with underweight, overweight, and obesity, *Journal of the American Medical Association* 2007; 298: 2028–37.

16. K. M. Flegal, M. D. Carroll, C. L. Ogden, and L. R. Curtin, Prevalence and trends in obesity among U.S. adults, 1999–2008, *Journal of the American Medical Association* 2010; 303: 235–41; C. L. Ogden, M. D. Carroll, L. R. Curtin, M. M. Lamb, and K. M. Flegal, Prevalence of high body mass index in U.S. children and adolescents, 2007–2008, *Journal of the American Medical Association* 2010; 303: 242–49.

17. See www.mskcc.org/aboutherbs.

18. See www.fda.gov.

19. I.-M. Lee, L. Djoussé, H. D. Sesso, L. Wang, and J. E. Buring, Physical activity and weight gain prevention, *Journal of the American Medical Association* 2010; 303: 1173–79.

20. S. N. Blair, J. B. Kampert, H. W. Kohl, et al., Influences of cardiorespiratory fitness and other precursors on cardiovascular disease and all-cause mortality in men and women, *Journal of the American Medical Association* 1996; 276: 205–10.

21. Physical Activity Guidelines Committee, *Physical activity guidelines advisory committee report* (Washington, D.C.: Department of Health and Human Services).

22. T. S. Church, C. P. Earnest, J. S. Skinner, and S. N. Blair, Effects of different doses of physical activity on cardiorespiratory fitness among sedentary, overweight or obese postmenopausal women with elevated blood pressure: A randomized controlled trial, *Journal of the American Medical Association* 2007; 297: 2081–91; I.-M. Lee, Dose-response relation between physical activity and fitness: Even a little is good; more is better, *Journal of the American Medical Association* 2007; 297: 2137–38.

23. T. E. Howe, L. Rochester, A. Jackson, P. M. H. Banks, and V. A. Blair, Exercise for improving balance in older people, Cochrane Database of Systematic Reviews 2007, issue 4, art. no. CD004963, doi:10.1002/14651858.CD004963.pub2; L. D. Gillespie, M. C. Robertson, W. J. Gillespie, et al., Interventions for preventing falls in elderly people, Cochrane Database of Systematic Reviews 2009, issue 2, art. no. CD007146, doi:10.1002/14651858. CD007146.pub2.

24. D. Bonaiuti, B. Shea, R. Iovine, et al., Exercise for preventing and treating osteoporosis in postmenopausal women, Cochrane Database of Systematic Reviews 2002, issue 2, art. no. CD000333, doi:10.1002/14651858.CD000333 (edited with no change in conclusions, issue 1, 2009); W. Kemmler, S. von Stengel, K. Engelke, L. Häberle, and W. A. Kalender, Exercise effects on bone mineral density, falls, coronary risk factors, and health care costs in older women, Archives of Internal Medicine 2010; 170: 179–85.

25. B. A. Lawton, S. B. Rose, C. R. Elley, et al., Exercise on prescription for women aged 40–74 recruited through primary care: Two year randomised controlled trial, British Medical Journal 2008; 337: a2509, doi:10.1136/bmj.a2509.

26. S. Ilffe, D. Kendrick, R. Morris, et al., Multi-centre cluster randomised trial comparing a community group exercise programme with home based exercise with usual care for people aged 65 and over in primary care: Protocol of the ProAct 65+ trial, Trials 2010; 11: 6–18.

27. A.-L. Kinmonth, N. I. Wareham, W. Hardeman, et al., Efficacy of a theory-based behavioural intervention to increase physical activity in an at-risk group in primary care (ProActive UK): A randomised trial, Lancet 2008; 371: 41–48.

28. S. K. Das, C. H. Gilhooly, J. K. Golden, et al., Long-term effects of 2 energy-restricted diets differing in glycemic load on dietary adherence, body composition and metabolism in CALERIE: A 1-y randomized controlled trial, American Journal of Clinical Nutrition 2007; 85: 1023–30; G. D. Foster, H. R. Wyatt, J. O. Hill, et al., Weight and metabolic outcomes after 2 years on a low-carbohydrate versus low-fat diet, Annals of Internal Medicine 2010; 153: 147–57.

29. G. M. Turner-McGrievy, N. D. Barnard, and A. R. Scialli, A two year randomized weight loss trial comparing a vegan diet to a more moderate low-fat diet, Obesity 2007; 15: 2276–81.

30. I. Shai, D. Schwarzfuchs, Y. Henkin, et al., Weight loss with a low-carbohydrate, Mediterranean-style diet, or low fat diet, New England Journal of Medicine 2008; 359: 229–41.

31. F. M. Sacks, G. A. Bray, V. J. Care, et al., Comparison of weight-loss diets with different compositions of fat, protein and carbohydrates, New England Journal of Medicine 2009; 360: 859–73; M. B. Katan, Weight-loss diets for the prevention and treatment of obesity, New England Journal of Medicine 2009; 360: 923–25.

32. P. W. Siri-Tarino, Q. Sun, F. B. Hu, and R. M. Krauss, Meta-analysis of prospective cohort studies evaluating the association of saturated fate with cardiovascular disease, American Journal of Clinical Nutrition, doi:10.3945/ajcn.2009.27725.

33. D. Rucker, R. Padwal, S. K. Ki, C. Curioni, and D. C. W. Lau, Long term pharmacotherapy for obesity and overweight: Updated meta-analysis, British Medical Journal 2007; doi:10:1136/bmj.39385.413113.25.

34. P. M. Ridker, E. Danielson, F. A. H. Fonseca, et al., Rosuvastatin to prevent vascular events in men and women with elevated C-reactive protein, *New England Journal of Medicine* 2008; 359, doi:10.1056/NEJMoa0807646

35. See http://abcnews.go.com/Health/HeartDiseaseNews/story?id=6207285&page=1.

36. G. Rose, *The strategy of preventive medicine* (New York: Oxford University Press, 1992).

37. S. Capewell, Will screening individuals at high risk of cardiovascular events deliver large benefits?, *British Medical Journal* 2008; 337: 785; M. S. Lauer, Primary prevention of atherosclerotic cardiovascular disease: The high public burden of low individual risk, *Journal of the American Medical Association* 2007; 297: 1376–78; K. K. Ray, S. R. K. Seshasai, S. Erqou, et al., Statins and all-cause mortality in high-risk primary prevention, *Archives of Internal Medicine* 2010; 170: 1024–31.

38. J. Lenzer, Truly independent research?, *British Medical Journal* 2008; 337: 602–6; M. de Lorgeril, P. Salen, J. Abramson, et al., Cholesterol lowering, cardiovascular diseases and rosuvastatin-JUPITER controversy, *Archives of Internal Medicine* 2010; 170: 1032–36.

39. D. Bassler, M. Briel, V. M. Montori, et al., Stopping randomized trials early for benefit and estimation of treatment effects: Systematic review and meta-regression analysis, *Journal of the American Medical Association* 2010; 303: 1180–87; S. Kaul, R. P. Morrissey, and G. A. Diamond, By Jove! What is a clinician to make of JUPITER?, *Archives of Internal Medicine* 2010; 170: 1073–76.

40. J. Hippisley-Cox and C. Coupland, Unintended effects of statins in men and women in England and Wales: Population based cohort study using the QResearch database, *British Medical Journal* 2010; 340: c2197, doi:10.1136/bjm.c2197.

41. P. M. Ridker, N. Rifai, L. Rose, et al., Comparison of C-reactive protein and low-density lipoprotein levels in the prediction of first cardiovascular events, *New England Journal of Medicine* 2002; 347: 1557–65; P. M. Ridker on behalf of the JUPITER Study Group, Rosuvastatin in the primary prevention of cardiovascular disease among patients with low levels of low-density lipoprotein cholesterol and elevated high-sensitivity C-reactive protein, *Circulation* 2003; 108: 2292–97.

42. P. Elliott, J. C. Chambers, W. Zhang, et al., Genetic loci associated with C-reactive protein levels and risk of coronary heart disease, *Journal of the American Medical Association* 2009; 302: 37–48; J. Zacho, A. Tybjærg-Hansen, J. S. Jensen, et al., Genetically elevated C-reactive protein and ischemic vascular disease, *New England Journal of Medicine* 2008; 359: 1897–908; H. Schunkert, N. J. Sarnani, Elevated C-reactive protein in atherosclerosis — chicken or egg?, *New England Journal of Medicine* 2008; 359: 1953–55.

43. I. Kushner, D. Samols, M. Magrey, A unifying biologic explanation for "High-Sensitivity" C-reactive protein and "Low-Grade" inflammation, *Arthritis Care and Research* 2010; 62: 442–46.

44. R. J. Glynn, W. Koenig, B. G. Nordestgaard, J. Shepherd, and P. M. Ridker, Rosuvastatin for primary prevention in older persons with elevated C-reactive protein and low to average low-density lipoprotein cholesterol levels: Exploratory analysis of a randomized trial, *Annals of Internal Medicine* 2010; 152: 488–96; S. J. Zieman and P. Ouyang, Statins for primary prevention in older adults: Who is at high risk, who is old and what denotes primary prevention?, *Annals of Internal Medicine* 2010; 152: 528–30.

45. A. Matheson, Corporate science and the husbandry of scientific and medical knowledge by the pharmaceutical industry, *BioSocieties* 2008; 3: 355–82; I. Boutron, S. Dutton, P. Ravaud, and D. G. Altman, Reporting and interpretation of randomized controlled trials with statistically nonsignificant results for primary outcomes, *Journal of the American Medical Association* 2010; 303: 2058–64; R. M. D. Smyth, J. J. Kirkham, A. Jacoby, et al., Frequency and reasons for outcome reporting bias in clinical trials: Interviews with trialists, *British Medical Journal* 2010; 341: e7151, doi:10.1136/BMJ.c7153.

46. M. Hochman, S. Hochman, D. Bor, and D. McCormick, News media coverage of medication research, *Journal of the American Medical Association* 2008; 300: 1544–50.

47. H. C. Sox and D. Rennie, Seeding trials: Just say "no," *Annals of Internal Medicine* 2008; 149: 279–80.

48. P. Slovic, M. Finucane, E. Peters, and D. G. MacGregor, Risk as analysis and risk as feelings: Some thoughts about affect, reason, risk and rationality, *Risk Analysis* 2004; 24: 1–12.

49. S. Woloshin, L. M. Schwartz, and H. G. Welch, The value of benefit data in direct-to-consumer drug ads, *Health Affairs* 2004 (Web exclusive, 28 April, W4–234).

50. U.S. Preventive Services Task Force, Screening for type 2 diabetes mellitus in adults: U.S. Preventive Services Task Force recommendation statement, *Annals of Internal Medicine* 2008; 148: 846–54.

51. University Group Diabetes Program (UGDP), A study of the effects of hypoglycemic agents on vascular complications in patients with adult-onset diabetes, *Diabetes* 1976; 25: 1129–53.

52. R. A. Whitmer, A. J. Karter, K. Yaffe, C. P. Quesenberry, and J. V. Selby, Hypoglycemic episodes and risk of dementia in older patients with type 2 diabetes mellitus, *Journal of the American Medical Association* 2009; 301: 1565–72.

53. R. Steinbrook, Facing the diabetes epidemic — Mandatory reporting of glycosylated hemoglobin values in New York City, *New England Journal of Medicine* 2006; 354: 545–48.

54. U. Bulugahapitiya, S. Siyambalapitiya, J. Sithole, and I. Idris, Is diabetes a coronary risk equivalent? Systematic review and meta-analysis, *Diabetes Medicine* 2009; 26: 142–48; The Emerging Risk Factors Collaboration, Diabetes mellitus, fasting blood glucose concentration, and risk of vascular disease: A collaborative meta-analysis of 102 prospective studies, *Lancet* 2010; 375: 2215–26.

55. J. Lindström, P. Ilanne Parikka, M. Peltonen, et al., Sustained reduction in the incidence of type 2 diabetes by lifestyle intervention: Follow-up of the Finnish Diabetes Prevention Study, *Lancet* 2006; 368: 1673–79; R. J. Sigal, G. P. Kenny, N. G. Boulé, et al., Effects of aerobic training, resistance training or both on glycemic control in type 2 diabetes, *Annals of Internal Medicine* 2007; 147: 357–69.

56. D. H. Solomon and W. C. Winkelmayer, Cardiovascular risk and the thiazolidinediones, *Journal of the American Medical Association* 2007; 298: 1216–18; S. Singh, Y. K. Loke, and C. D. Furberg, Long-term risk of cardiovascular events with rosiglitazone: A meta-analysis, *Journal of the American Medical Association* 2007; 298: 1189–95; A. M. Lincoff, K. Wolski, S. J. Nicholls, and S. E. Nissen, Pioglitazone and risk of cardiovascular events in patients with type 2 diabetes mellitus: A meta-analysis of randomized trials, *Journal of the American Medical Association* 2007; 298: 1180–88.

57. L. L. Lipscombe, T. Gomes, L. E. Lévesque, et al., Thiazolidinediones and cardiovascular outcomes in older patients with diabetes, *Journal of the American Medical Association* 2007; 298: 2634–43.

58. S. E. Nissen and K. Wolski, Effect of rosiglitazone on the risk of myocardial infarction and death from cardiovascular causes, *New England Journal of Medicine* 2007; 356: 2457–71.

59. J. M. Drazen, S. Morrissey, and G. D. Curfman, Rosiglitazone—Continued uncertainty about safety, *New England Journal of Medicine* 2007: 357: 63–64; D. M. Nathan, Rosiglitazone and cardiotoxicity—Weighing the evidence, *New England Journal of Medicine* 2007; 357: 64–66; B. M. Psaty and C. D. Furberg, Rosiglitazone and cardiovascular risk, *New England Journal of Medicine* 2007; 356: 2522–24.

60. C. J. Rosen, The rosiglitazone story—Lessons from an FDA advisory committee meeting, *New England Journal of Medicine* 2007; 357: 844–46; U.S. Food and Drug Administration 2007, www.fda.gov/medwatch/safety/2007/safety07.htm#rosi_pio; European Medicines Agency, Questions and answers on the benefits and risks of rosiglitazone and pioglitazone, 2007, www.emea.europa.eu/pdfs/human/press/pr/48446407en.pdf.

61. P. D. Home, S. J. Pocock, H. Beck-Nielson, et al., Rosiglitazone evaluated for cardiac outcomes—An interim analysis, *New England Journal of Medicine* 2007; 357: 28–38.

62. B. M. Psaty and C. D. Furberg, The record on rosiglitazone and the risk of myocardial infarction, *New England Journal of Medicine* 2007; 357: 67–69.

63. S. E. Nissen, Setting the RECORD straight, *Journal of the American Medical Association* 2010; 303: 1194–95.

64. C. D. De Angelis and P. B. Fontanarosa, Ensuring integrity in industry-sponsored research, *Journal of the American Medical Association* 2010; 303: 1196–98; Staff report on GlaxoSmithKline and the Diabetes Drug Avandia prepared by the staff of the Committee on Finance, U.S. Senate, http://finance.senate.gov/press/Gpress/2010/prg022010a.pdf.

65. J. H. Tanne, GSK is accused of trying to suppress editorial on rosiglitazone, *British Medical Journal* 2010; 340: c2654; S. E. Nissen, The rise and fall of rosiglitazone, *European Heart Journal* 2010; 31: 773–76.

66. K. K. Ray, S. R. Seshasai, S. Wijesuriya, et al., Effect of intensive control of glucose on cardiovascular outcomes and death in patients with diabetes mellitus: A meta-analysis of randomised controlled trials, *Lancet* 2009; 373: 1765–72; W. Duckworth, C. Abraira, T. Moritz, et al., Glucose control and vascular complications in veterans with type 2 diabetes, *New England Journal of Medicine* 2009; 360: 129–39; T. N. Kelly, L. A. Bazzano, V. A. Fonseca, et al., Systematic review: Glucose control and cardiovascular disease in type 2 diabetes, *Annals of Internal Medicine* 2009; 151: 394–403.

67. The ADVANCE Collaborative Group, Intensive blood glucose control and vascular outcomes in patients with type 2 diabetes, *New England Journal of Medicine* 2008; 358: 2560–72; M. Mitka, Aggressive glycemic control might not be best choice for all diabetic patients, *Journal of the American Medical Association* 2010; 303: 1137–38.

68. H. W. Rodbard, P. S. Jellinger, J. A. Davidson, et al., Statement by an American Association of Clinical Endocrinologists/American College of Endocrinology consensus panel on type 2 diabetes mellitus: An algorithm for glycemic control, *Endocrine Practice* 2009; 15: 541–59.

69. American Diabetes Association, Executive summary: Standards of medical care in diabetes—2009, *Diabetes Care* 2009; 32 (supplement 1): S6–12.

70. A. T. Wang, C. P. McCoy, M. H. Murah, and V. M. Monton, Association between industry affiliation and position on cardiovascular risk with rosiglitazone: Cross sectional systematic review, *British Medical Journal* 2010; 340: c1344, doi:10.1136/bmj.c1344.

71. N. M. Hadler, Ethics Forum: Would physician disclosure of all industry gifts solve the conflict-of-interest problem? Negative Constructive, *American Medical (AMA) News*, January 7, 2008.

72. Nissen, Setting the RECORD straight.

73. ACCORD Study Group, Effects of intensive blood-pressure control in type 2 diabetes mellitus, *New England Journal of Medicine* 2010; 362: 1575–85.

74. ACCORD Study Group, Effects of combination lipid therapy in type 2 diabetes mellitus, *New England Journal of Medicine* 2010; 362: 1563–74.

75. M. O. Goodarzi and B. M. Psaty, Glucose lowering to control macrovascular disease in type 2 diabetes, *Journal of the American Medical Association* 2008; 300: 2051–53.

76. A. D. Rule, H. Amer, L. D. Cornell, et al., The association between age and nephrosclerosis on renal biopsy among healthy adults, *Annals of Internal Medicine* 2010; 152: 561–67.

77. B. M. Egan, Y. Zhao, and R. N. Axon, U.S. trends in prevalence, awareness, treatment, and control of hypertension, 1988–2008, *Journal of the American Medical Association* 2010; 303: 2043–50.

78. R. S. Vasan, M. G. Larson, E. P. Leip, et al., Impact of high-normal blood pressure on the risk of cardiovascular disease, *New England Journal of Medicine* 2001; 345: 1291–97; S. Port, L. Demer, R. Jennrich, D. Walter, and A. Garfinkel, Systolic blood pressure and mortality, *Lancet* 2000; 35: 175–80.

79. U.S. Preventive Services Task Force, Screening for high blood pressure: U.S. Preventive Services Task Force reaffirmation recommendation statement, *Annals of Internal Medicine* 2007; 147: 783–86; T. Wolff and T. Miller, Evidence for the reaffirmation of the U.S. Preventive Services Task Force recommendation on screening for high blood pressure, *Annals of Internal Medicine* 2007; 147: 787–91.

80. M. R. Law, J. K. Morris, and N. J. Wald, Use of blood pressure lowering drugs in the prevention of cardiovascular disease: Meta-analysis of 147 randomised trials in the context of expectations from prospective epidemiological studies, *British Medical Journal* 2009; 338: b1665, doi:10.1136/bmj.b1665.

81. See note 45 of this chapter.

82. Multiple Risk Intervention Trial Research Group, Multiple Risk Factor Intervention Trial: Risk factor changes and mortality, *Journal of the American Medical Association* 1982; 248: 182–87.

83. J. T. Wright, J. L. Probstfield, W. C. Cushman, et al., ALLHAT findings revisited in the context of subsequent analyses, other trials, and meta-analyses, *Archives of Internal Medicine* 2009; 169: 832–42.

84. G. Davey Smith, J. D. Neaton, D. Wentworth, et al., Mortality differences between black and white men in the USA: Contribution of income and other risk factors among men screened for the MR FIT, *Lancet* 1998; 351: 934–39.

85. J. M. Wright and V. M. Musini, First-line drugs for hypertension, Cochrane Database of Systematic Reviews 2009 issue 3, art. no. CD001841, doi:10.1002/14651858.CD001841. pub2.

86. F. M. Sacks and H. Campos, Dietary therapy in hypertension, *New England Journal of Medicine* 2010; 362: 2102–12; L. J. Appel and C. A. M. Anderson, Compelling evidence for public health action to reduce salt intake, *New England Journal of Medicine* 2010; 362: 650–52; T. Frieden and P. A. Briss, We can reduce dietary sodium, save money and save lives, *Annals of Internal Medicine* 2010; 152: 526–27

87. M. H. Alderman, Reducing dietary sodium: The case for caution, *Journal of the American Medical Association* 2010; 303: 448–49.

88. A. V. Chobanian, Does it matter how hypertension is controlled?, *New England Journal of Medicine* 2008; 359: 2485–88.

89. I. Boger-Megiddo, S. R. Heckbert, N. S. Weiss, et al., Myocardial infarction and stroke associated with diuretic based two drug antihypertensive regimens: Population based case-control study, *British Medical Journal* 2010; 340: c103, doi:10.1136/bmj.c103.

90. J. A. Arguedas, M. I. Perez, and J. M. Wright, Treatment blood pressure targets for hypertension, Cochrane Database of Systematic Reviews 2009, issue 3, art. no. CD004349, doi:10.1002/14651858.CD004349.pub2.

91. Blood Pressure Lowering Treatment Trialists' Collaboration, Effects of different regimens to lower blood pressure on major cardiovascular events in older and younger people: Meta-analysis of randomised trials, *British Medical Journal* 2008; doi:10.1136/bmj.39548.738368.BE.

92. R. M. Cooper-DeHolt, Y. Gong, and E. M. Handberg, et al., Tight blood pressure control and cardiovascular outcomes among hypertensive patients with diabetes and coronary artery disease, *Journal of the American Medical Association* 2010; 304: 61–68.

93. H. M. Perry, B. R. Davis, T. R. Price, et al., Effect of treating isolated systolic hypertension on the risk of developing various types and subtypes of stroke, *Journal of the American Medical Association* 2000; 284: 465–71; S. Lewington, R. Clarke, N. Qizilbash, R. Peto, and R. Collins, Prospective Studies Collaboration, Age-specific relevance of usual blood pressure to vascular mortality: A meta-analysis of individual data for one million adults in 61 prospective studies, *Lancet* 2002; 360: 1903–13.

94. J. B. Kostis, Treating hypertension in the very old, *New England Journal of Medicine* 2008; 358: 1958–60.

95. H. C. Wijeysundera, M. Machado, F. Farahati, et al., Association of temporal trends in risk factors and treatment uptake with coronary heart disease mortality, 1994–2005, *Journal of the American Medical Association* 2010; 303: 1841–47.

96. L. Byberg, H. Melhus, R. Gedeborg, et al., Total mortality after changes in leisure time physical activity in 50 year old men: 35 year follow-up of population based cohort, *British Medical Journal* 2009; 338: b688, doi:10.1136/bmj.b688.

97. S. Stringhini, S. Sabia, M. Shipley, et al., Association of socioeconomic position with health behaviors and mortality, *Journal of the American Medical Association* 2010; 303: 1159–66; E. Kvaavik, D. Batty, G. Ursin, R. Huxley, and C. R. Gale, Influence of individual and combined health behaviors on total and cause-specific mortality in men and women, *Archives of Internal Medicine* 2010; 170: 711–18.

98. M. O'Flaherty, J. Bishop, A. Redpath, et al., Coronary heart disease mortality among

young adults in Scotland in relation to social inequalities: Time trend study, *British Medical Journal* 2009; 338: b2613, doi:10.1136/bmj.b2613.

99. A. H. Leyland and J. W. Lynch, Why has mortality from coronary heart disease in young adults leveled off?, *British Medical Journal* 2009; 338: b2515, doi:10.1136/bmj.b2515.

100. H. M. Krumholz, Y. Wang, J. Chen, et al., Reduction in acute myocardial infarction mortality in the United States: Risk-standardized mortality rates from 1995–2006, *Journal of the American Medical Association* 2009; 302: 767–73; R. W. Yeh, S. Sidney, M. Chandra, et al., Population trends in the incidence and outcomes of acute myocardial infarction, *New England Journal of Medicine* 2010; 362: 2155–65.

101. R. A. Henderson, S. J. Pocock, T. C. Clayton, et al., Seven-year outcome in the RITA-2 trial: Coronary angioplasty versus medical therapy, *Journal of the American College of Cardiology* 2003; 42: 1161–70.

102. M. Pfisterer, P. Buser, S. Osswald, et al., Outcome of elderly patients with chronic symptomatic coronary artery disease with an invasive vs. optimized medical treatment strategy, *Journal of the American Medical Association* 2003; 289: 1117–23.

103. W. E. Boden, R. A. O'Rourke, K. K. Teo, et al., Optimal medical therapy with or without PCI for stable coronary disease, *New England Journal of Medicine* 2007; 336: 1503–16.

104. J. S. Hochman, G. A. Lamas, C. E. Buller, et al., Coronary intervention for persistent occlusion after myocardial infarction, *New England Journal of Medicine* 2006; 355: 2395–407.

105. BARI 2D Study Group, A randomized trial of therapies for type 2 diabetes and coronary artery disease, *New England Journal of Medicine* 2009; 360: 2503–15.

106. H. C. Wijeysundera, B. K. Nallamothu, H. M. Krumholz, J. V. Tu, and D. T. Ko, Meta-analysis: Effects of percutaneous coronary intervention versus medical therapy on angina relief, *Annals of Internal Medicine* 2010; 152: 370–79; B. K. Nallamothu and H. M. Krumholz, Putting ad hoc PCI on pause, *Journal of the American Medical Association* 2010; 304: 2059–60.

107. Antithrombotic Trialists' Collaboration, Aspirin in the primary and secondary prevention of vascular disease. Collaborative meta analysis of individual participant data from randomised trials, *Lancet* 2009; 373: 1849–60.

108. See http://www.businessweek.com/technology/content/jul2005/tc2005077_3265_tc024.htm.

109. P. Meier, G. Knapp, U. Tamhane, S. Chaturvedi, and H. S. Gurm, Short term and intermediate term comparison of endarectomy versus stenting for carotid artery stenosis: Systematic review and meta-analysis of randomised controlled clinical trials, *British Medical Journal* 2010; 340: c467, doi:10.1136/bmj.c467; T. G. Brott, R. W. Hobson, G. Howard, et al., Stenting versus endarterectomy for treatment of carotid-artery stenosis, *New England Journal of Medicine* 2010; 363: 11–23.

110. L. Bax, A.-J. J. Woittiez, H. J. Kouwenberg, et al., Stent placement in patients with atherosclerotic renal artery stenosis and impaired renal function, *Annals of Internal Medicine* 2009; 150: 840–48.

111. The United Kingdom EVAR Trial Investigators, Endovascular versus open repair of abdominal aortic aneurysm, *New England Journal of Medicine* 2010; 362: 1863–71.

112. K. C. Kent, Endovascular aneurysm repair—Is it durable?, *New England Journal of Medicine* 2010; 162: 1930–31.

113. N. M. Hadler, A ripe old age, *Archives of Internal Medicine* 2003; 163: 1261–62.

114. E. Boulware, S. Marinopoulos, K. A. Phillips, et al., Systematic review: The value of the periodic health evaluation, *Annals of Internal Medicine* 2007; 146: 289–300.

Chapter 3

1. L. Esserman, Y. Shieh, and I. Thompson, Rethinking screening for breast cancer and prostate cancer, *Journal of the American Medical Association* 2009; 302: 1685–92.

2. U.S. Preventive Services Task Force, Screening for breast cancer: U.S. Preventive Services Task Force recommendation statement, *Annals of Internal Medicine* 2009; 151: 716–26.

3. J. S. Mandelblatt, K. A. Cronin, S. Bailey, et al., Effects of mammography screening under different screening schedules: Model estimates of potential benefits and harms, *Annals of Internal Medicine* 2009; 151: 738–47.

4. A. N. A. Tosteson, N. K. Stout, D. G. Fryback, et al., Cost-effectiveness of digital mammography breast cancer screening, *Annals of Internal Medicine* 2008; 148: 1–10.

5. H. D. Nelson, K. Tyne, A. Naik, et al., Screening for breast cancer: An update for the U.S. Preventive Services Task Force, *Annals of Internal Medicine* 2009; 151: 727–37.

6. K.-A. Phillip, G. Glendon, and J. A. Knight, Putting the risk of breast cancer in perspective, *New England Journal of Medicine* 1999; 340: 141–44.

7. N. M. Hadler, *Worried sick: A prescription for health in an overtreated America* (Chapel Hill: University of North Carolina Press, 2008).

8. Nelson, Tyne, Naik, et al., Screening for breast cancer.

9. O. S. Miettinen, C. T. Henschke, M. W. Pasmantler, et al., Does mammography save lives?, *Canadian Medical Association Journal* 2002; 166: 1187–88; O. S. Miettinen, C. T. Henschke, M. W. Pasmantler, et al., Mammographic screening: No reliable supporting evidence?, *Lancet* 2002; 359: 404–6.

10. J. P. Kösters and P. C. Gøtzsche, Regular self-examination or clinical examination for early detection of breast cancer, Cochrane Database of Systematic Reviews 2003, issue 2, art. no. CD003373, doi:10.1002/14651858.CD003373. This version first published online on April 22, 2003; last assessed as up-to-date on October 9, 2007.

11. T. Hampton, Oncologists advise breast awareness over routine breast self-examination, *Journal of the American Medical Association* 2008; 300: 1748–49.

12. See Hadler, *Worried sick*; N. M. Hadler, *The last well person: How to stay well despite the health-care system* (Montreal: McGill-Queens University Press, 2004).

13. Esserman, Shieh, and Thompson, Rethinking screening for breast cancer and prostate cancer.

14. See http://www.peoplespharmacy.com/2009/11/07/747-health-news-update/.

15. R. D. Truog, Screening mammography and the "R" word, *New England Journal of Medicine* 2009; 361: 2501–3.

16. J. Crewdson, Rethinking the mammogram guidelines, *Atlantic Monthly*, November 19, 2009.

17. L. M. Schwartz and S. Woloshin, Participation in mammography screening: Women should be encouraged to decide what is right for them, rather than being told what to do, *British Medical Journal* 2007; 335: 731–32.

18. N. T. Brewer, T. Salz, and S. E. Lillie, Systematic review: The long-term effects of false-positive mammograms, *Annals of Internal Medicine* 2007; 146: 502–10.

19. K. Armstrong, E. Moye, S. Williams, et al., Screening mammography in women 40 to 49 years of age: A systematic review for the American College of Physicians, *Annals of Internal Medicine* 2007; 146: 516–26; A. Berrington de Gonzalez, C. D. Berg, K. Visvanathan, and M. Robson, Estimated risk of radiation-induced breast cancer from mammographic screening for young BRCA mutation carriers, *Journal of the National Cancer Institute* 2009; 101: 205–9.

20. P.-H. Zahl, J. Mæhlen, and H. G. Welch, The natural history of invasive breast cancers detected by screening mammography, *Archives of Internal Medicine* 2008; 168: 2311–16.

21. K. J. Jørgensen and P. Gøtzsche, Overdiagnosis in publicly organized mammography screening programmes: Systematic review of incidence trends, *British Medical Journal* 2009; 339: b2587.

22. H. G. Welch, Overdiagnosis and mammography screening: The question is no longer whether, but how often it occurs, *British Medical Journal* 2009; 339: 182–83; H. G. Welch, Screening mammography—A long run for a short slide, *New England Journal of Medicine* 2010; 363: 1276–78.

23. Esserman, Shieh, and Thompson, Rethinking screening for breast cancer and prostate cancer.

24. S. Woloshin and L. M. Schwartz, The benefits and harms of mammography screening: Understanding the trade-offs, *Journal of the American Medical Association* 2010; 303: 164–65; H. G. Welch, L. M. Schwartz, and S. Woloshin, *Over-diagnosed* (Boston: Beacon Press, 2011).

25. Q. Deeley, The cognitive anthropology of belief, in *The power of belief: Psychosocial influences on illness, disability, and medicine*, ed. P. W. Halligan and M. Aylward (Oxford: Oxford University Press, 2006), 33–54.

26. I. Hacking, *The social construction of what?* (Cambridge: Harvard University Press, 1999).

27. N. M. Hadler, *Stabbed in the back: Confronting back pain in an overtreated society* (Chapel Hill: University of North Carolina Press, 2009).

28. S. Sontag, *Illness as metaphor* (New York, Farrar Straus and Giroux, 1978).

29. L. M. Schwartz, S. Woloshin, F. J. Fowler, and H. G. Welch, Enthusiasm for cancer screening in the United States, *Journal of the American Medical Association* 2004; 291: 71–78.

30. M. E. Young, G. R. Norman, and K. R. Humphreys, The role of medical language in changing public perceptions of illness, *PLoS One* 2008; 3: e3875–80.

31. K. Finkler, *Experiencing the new genetics: Family and kinship on the medical frontier* (Philadelphia: University of Pennsylvania Press, 2000).

32. L. M. Schwartz, S. Woloshin, E. I. Dvorin, and H. G. Welch, Ratio measures in leading medical journals: Structured review of accessibility of underlying absolute risks, *British Medical Journal*, doi:10.1136/bmj.38985.564317.7C (published 23 October 2006).

33. P. C. Gøtzsche, Believability of relative risks and odds ratios in abstracts: Cross sectional study, *British Medical Journal* 2006; 333: 231–34.

34. S. Woloshin, L. M. Schwartz, S. L. Casella, A. T. Kennedy, and R. J. Larson, Press

releases by academic medical centers: Not so academic?, *Annals of Internal Medicine* 209; 150: 613–18.

35. American College of Obstetricians and Gynecologists, Cervical cytology screening, ACOG Practice Bulletin no. 109 (December 2009), published in *Obstetrics and Gynecology* 2009; 14: 1409–20.

36. M. Kyrgiou, G. Koliopoulos, P. Martin-Hirsch, M. Arbyn, W. Prendiville, and E. Paraskevaidis, Obstetric outcomes after conservative treatment for intraepithelial or early invasive cervical lesions: Systematic review and meta-analysis, *Lancet* 2006; 367: 489–98.

37. G. F. Sawaya, Cervical-cancer screening—New guidelines and the balance between benefits and harms, *New England Journal of Medicine* 2009; 361: 2503–5.

38. M. R. E. McCredie, K. J. Sharples, C. Paul, J. Baranyai, et al., Natural history of cervical neoplasia and risk of invasive cancer in women with cervical intraepithelial neoplasia 3: A retrospective cohort study, *Lancet* 2008; 9: 425–34.

39. P. T. Scardino, Localized prostate cancer is rarely a fatal disease, *Nature Clinical Practice Urology* 2008; 5: 1 (PMID: 18185510).

40. M. J. Barry and A. J. Mulley, Why are a high overdiagnosis probability and a long lead time for prostate cancer screening so important?, *Journal of the National Cancer Institute* 2009; 101: 362–63.

41. A. L. Potosky, B. A. Miller, P. C. Albertsen, and B. S. Kramer, The role of increasing determination in the rising incidence of prostate cancer, *Journal of the American Medical Association* 1995; 273: 548–52.

42. L. E. Ross, Z. Berkowitz, and D. U. Ekwueme, Use of the prostate-specific antigen test among U.S. men: Findings from the 2005 National Health Interview Survey, *Cancer Epidemiology Biomarkers and Prevention* 2008; 17: 636–44.

43. E. C. Chan, M. J. Barry, S. W. Vernon, and C. Ahn, Brief report: Physicians and their personal prostate cancer-screening practices with prostate-specific antigen, *Journal of General Internal Medicine* 2006; 21: 257–59.

44. Hadler, *Worried sick*; Hadler, *The last well person*.

45. U.S. Preventive Services Task Force, Screening for prostate cancer: U.S. Preventive Services Task Force recommendation statement, *Annals of Internal Medicine* 2008; 149: 185–91; K. Lin, R. Lipsitz, T. Miller, and S. Janakiraman, Benefits and harms of prostate-specific antigen screening for prostate cancer: An evidence update for the U.S. Preventive Services Task Force, *Annals of Internal Medicine* 2008; 149: 192–99.

46. See www.auanet.org.

47. M. Mitka, Urology group: Prostate screening should be offered beginning at age 40, *Journal of the American Medical Association* 2009; 301: 2538–39.

48. K. Fall, F. Fang, L. A. Mucci, et al., Immediate risk for cardiovascular events and suicide following a prostate cancer diagnosis: Prospective cohort study, *PLoS Medicine* 2009; 6 (12): e1000197.

49. D. P. Smith, M. T. King, S. Egger, et al., Quality of life three years after diagnosis of localised prostate cancer: Population based cohort study, *British Medical Journal* 2009; 339: b4817, doi:10.1136/bmj.b4817.

50. G. L. Andriole, R. L. Grubb, S. S. Buys, et al., Mortality results from a randomized prostate-cancer screening trial, *New England Journal of Medicine* 2009; 360: 1310–19.

51. F. H. Schröder, J. Hugosson, M. J. Roobol, et al., Screening and prostate-cancer mortality in a randomized European study, *New England Journal of Medicine* 2009; 360: 1320–28.

52. B. Holmström, M. Johansson, A. Bergh, et al., Prostate specific antigen for early detection of prostate cancer: Longitudinal study, *British Medical Journal* 2009; 339: b3537, doi:10:1136/bjm.b3537; M. Djulbegovic, R. Beyth, M. M. Neuberger, T. L. Stoffs, J. Vieweg, B. Djulbegovic, and P. Dahm, Screening for prostate cancer: Systematic review and meta-analysis of randomized controlled trials, *British Medical Journal* 2010; 341: c4543, doi:10.1136/bmj.c4543; J. H. Hayes, D. A. Ollendorf, S. D. Pearson, et al., Active surveillance compared with initial treatment for men with low-risk prostate cancer, *Journal of the American Medical Association* 2010; 304: 2372–80.

53. E. P. Gelmann and S. M. Henshall, Clinically relevant prognostic markers for prostate cancer: The search goes on, *Annals of Internal Medicine* 2009; 150: 647–49.

54. N. N. Baxter, M. A. Goldwasser, L. F. Paszat, R. Saskin, D. R. Urbach, and L. Rabeneck, Association of colonoscopy and death from colorectal cancer, *Annals of Internal Medicine* 2009; 150: 1–8.

55. J. L. Warren, C. N. Klabunde, A. B. Mariotto, et al., Adverse events after outpatient colonoscopy in the Medicare population, *Annals of Internal Medicine* 2009; 150: 849–57.

56. N. M. Gatto, H. Frucht, V. Sundararajan, J. S. Jacobson, V. R. Grann, and A. I. Neugut, Risk of perforation after colonoscopy and sigmoidoscopy: A population based study, *Journal of the National Cancer Institute* 2003; 95: 230–36.

57. B. Bressler, L. F. Paszat, Z. Chen, et al., Rates of new or missed colorectal cancers after colonoscopy and their risk factors: A population-based analysis, *Gastroenterology* 2007; 132: 96–102.

58. R. L. Barclay, J. J. Vicari, A. S. Doughty, J. F. Johanson, and R. L. Greenlaw, Colonoscopic withdrawal times and adenoma detection during screening colonoscopy, *New England Journal of Medicine* 2006; 355: 2533–41.

59. D. F. Ransohoff, How much does colonoscopy reduce colon cancer mortality?, *Annals of Internal Medicine* 2009; 150: 50–52.

60. G. Hoff, T. Grotmoi, E. Skovlund, and M. Bretthauer for the Norwegian Colorectal Cancer Prevention Study Group, Risk of colorectal cancer seven years after flexible sigmoidoscopy screening: Randomised controlled trial, *British Medical Journal* 2009; 338: b1846.

61. T. F. Imperiale, Sigmoidoscopy screening for colorectal cancer, *British Medical Journal* 2009; 338: b2084, doi:10.1136/bmj.b2084.

62. W. S. Atkin, R. Edwards, I. Kralj-Hans, et al., Once-only flexible sigmoidoscopy screening in prevention of colorectal cancer: A multicentre randomised controlled trial, *Lancet* 2010; 375: 1624–33; D. Ransohoff, Can endoscopy protect against colorectal cancer? An RCT, *Lancet* 2010; 375: 1582–84.

63. T. F. Imperiale, E. A. Glowinski, C. Lin-Cooper, G. N. Larkin, J. D. Rogge, and D. F. Ransohoff, Five-year risk of colorectal neoplasia after negative screening colonoscopy, *New England Journal of Medicine* 2008; 359: 1218–24.

64. M. Pignone and H. C. Sox, Screening guidelines for colorectal cancer: A twice-told tale, *Annals of Internal Medicine* 2008; 149: 680–82.

65. See www.ahrq.gov/clinic/uspstfix.htm.

66. J. Guirguis-Blake, N. Calonge, T. Miller, A. Siu, S. Teutsch, and E. Whitlock, Current processes of the U.S. Preventive Services Task Force: Refining evidence-based recommendation development, *Annals of Internal Medicine* 2007; 147: 117–22; M. B. Barton, T. Miller, T. Wolff, et al., How to read the new recommendation statement: Methods update from the U.S. Preventive Services Task Force, *Annals of Internal Medicine* 2007; 147: 123–27.

67. E. P. Whitlock, J. S. Lin, E. Liles, T. L. Beil, and R. Fu, Screening for colorectal cancer: A targeted, updated systematic review for the U.S. Preventive Services Task Force, *Annals of Internal Medicine* 2008; 149: 638–58.

68. A. G. Zauber, I. Lansdorp-Vogelaar, A. Knudsen, J. Wilschut, M. van Ballegooijen, and K. M. Kuntz, Evaluating test strategies for colorectal cancer screening: A decision analysis for the U.S. Preventive Services Task Force, *Annals of Internal Medicine* 2008; 149: 659–69.

69. B. Levin, D. A. Lieberman, B. McFarland, et al., American Cancer Society Colorectal Cancer Advisory Group, U.S. Multi-Society Task Force, American College of Radiology Colon Cancer Committee, Screening and surveillance for the early detection of colorectal cancer and adenomatous polyps, 2008: A joint guideline from the American Cancer Society, the U.S. Multi-Society Task Force on Colorectal Cancer, and the American College of Gastroenterology, *Gastroenterology* 2008; 134: 1570–95.

70. D. A. Lieberman, Screening for colorectal cancer, *New England Journal of Medicine* 2009; 361: 1179–87.

71. H. K. Roy and L. K. Bianchi, Differences in colon adenomas and carcinomas among women and men, *Journal of the American Medical Association* 2009; 302: 1696–97.

72. N. K. Choudry, H. T. Stelfox, and A. S. Detsky, Relationships between authors of clinical practice guidelines and the pharmaceutical industry, *Journal of the American Medical Association* 2002; 287: 612–17.

73. P. Tricoci, J. M. Allen, J. M. Kramer, et al., Scientific evidence underlying the ACC/AHA clinical practice guidelines, *Journal of the American Medical Association* 2009; 301: 831–41.

74. A. S. Detsky, Sources for bias for authors of clinical practice guidelines, *Canadian Medical Association Journal* 2006; 175: 1033–35; T. M. Shaneyfelt and R. M. Centor, Reassessment of clinical practice guidelines, *Journal of the American Medical Association* 2009; 301: 868–69.

75. S. D. Markowitz and M. M. Bertagnolli, Molecular basis of colorectal cancer, *New England Journal of Medicine* 2009; 361: 2449–60.

76. Hadler, *Worried sick*.

77. M. Schermerhorn, A 66-year-old man with an abdominal aortic aneurysm: Review of screening and treatment, *Journal of the American Medical Association* 2009; 302: 2015–22; M. L. Schermerhorn, A. J. O'Maley, A. Jhaveri, et al., Endovascular vs. open repair of abdominal aortic aneurysms in the Medicare population, *New England Journal of Medicine* 2008; 358: 464–74.

78. N. M. Hadler, A ripe old age, *Archives of Internal Medicine* 2003; 163: 1261–62.

79. S. H. Thompson, H. A. Ashton, L. Gao, R. A. P. Scott, Multicentre Aneurysm Screening Group, Screening men for abdominal aortic aneurysm: 10 year mortality and cost effectiveness results from the randomised Multicentre Aneurysm Screening Study, *British Medical Journal* 2009; 338: b2307.

80. L. Ehlers, K. Overvad, J. Sørensen, et al., Analysis of cost effectiveness of screening Danish men aged 65 for abdominal aortic aneurysm, *British Medical Journal* 2009; 338: b2243.

81. R. M. Leipzig, E. P. Whitlock, T. A. Wolff, et al., Reconsidering the approach to prevention recommendations for older adults, *Annals of Internal Medicine* 2010; 153: 809–14; M. E. Tinetti, Making prevention recommendations relevant for an aging population, *Annals of Internal Medicine* 2010; 153: 843–44.

82. V. Entwistle, Communicating about screening, *British Medical Journal* 2008; 337: 789–91; The trouble with screening (editorial), *Lancet* 2009; 373: 1223.

Chapter 4

1. E. H. Ackernecht, *Rudolf Virchow* (Madison: University of Wisconsin Press, 1953).

2. K. C. Volpp, W. Friedman, P. J. Romano, et al., Residency training at a crossroads: Duty-hour standards 2010, *Annals of Internal Medicine* 2010; 153: 826–28.

3. U.S. General Accounting Office, *Older workers: Policies of other nations to increase labor force participation* (Washington, D.C.: U.S. General Accounting Office, 2003).

4. M. D. Giandrea, K. E. Cahill, and J. F. Quinn, *Self-employment transitions among older American workers with career jobs*, BLS Working Paper 418, April 2008 (www.bls .gov/osmr/pdf/ec080040.pdf).

5. N. M. Hadler, *Stabbed in the back: Confronting back pain in an overtreated society* (Chapel Hill: University of North Carolina Press, 2009).

6. C. Bamia, A. Trichopoulou, and D. Trichopoulos, Age at retirement and mortality in a general population sample: The Greek EPIC study, *American Journal of Epidemiology* 2007; 167: 561–69.

7. I. Kawachi and L. Berkman, Social cohesion, social capital, and health, chapter 8 of *Social Epidemiology*, ed. L. Berkman and I. Kawachi (Oxford: Oxford University Press, 2000), 174–90.

8. I. Kawachi, B. P. Kennedy, K. Lochner, and D. Prothrow-Stith, Social capital, income inequality and mortality, *American Journal of Public Health* 1997; 87: 1491–98.

9. M. Marmot, *The Status Syndrome: How social standing affects our health and longevity* (New York: Henry Holt, 2004).

10. R. Karasek and T. Theorell, *Healthy work: Stress, productivity, and the reconstruction of working life* (New York: Basic Books, 1990).

11. K. E. Cahill, M. D. Giandrea, and J. F. Quinn, Retirement patterns from career employment, *Gerontologist* 2006; 46: 514–23.

12. S. Ferlander, The importance of different forms of social capital for health, *Acta Sociologica* 2007; 50: 115–28.

13. M. J. De Silva, K. McKenzie, T. Harpham, et al., Social capital and mental illness: A systematic review, *Journal of Epidemiology and Community Health* 2005; 59: 619–27.

14. A. Kouvonen, T. Oksanen, J. Vahtera, et al., Low workplace social capital as a predictor of depression: The Finnish Public Sector Study, *American Journal of Epidemiology* 2008; 167: 1143–51.

15. A. Väänänen, A. Kouvonen, M. Kivimäki, et al., Workplace social capital and co-occurrence of lifestyle risk factors: The Finnish Public Sector Study, *Journal of Occupa-*

tional and Environmental Medicine 2009; 66: 432–37; A. L. Sapp, I. Kawachi, G. Sorensen, A. D. LaMontagne, and S. V. Subramanian, Does workplace social capital buffer the effects of job stress? A cross-sectional, multilevel analysis of cigarette smoking among U.S. manufacturing workers, *Journal of Occupational and Environmental Health* 2010; 52: 740–50.

16. T. Oksanen, A. Kouvonen, J. Vahtera, et al., Prospective study of workplace social capital and depression: Are vertical and horizontal components equally important?, *Journal of Epidemiology and Community Health*, 19 August 2009, doi:10.1136/jech.2008.086074.

17. M. Lindström and the Malmö Shoulder-Neck Study Group, Psychosocial work conditions, social participation and social capital: A causal pathway investigated in a longitudinal study, *Social Science and Medicine* 2006; 62: 280–91.

18. Karasek and Theorell, *Healthy work*.

19. R. Rugulies, B. Aust, J. Siegrist, et al., Distribution of effort-reward imbalance in Denmark and its prospective association with a decline in self-rated health, *Journal of Occupational and Environmental Health* 2009; 51: 870–78.

20. E. B. Faragher, M. Cass, and C. L. Cooper, The relationship between job satisfaction and health: A meta-analysis, *Journal of Occupational and Environmental Medicine* 2005; 62: 105–21.

21. D. O'Reilly, M. Rosato, and C. Patterson, Self reported health and mortality: Ecological analysis based on electoral wards across the United Kingdom, *British Medical Journal* 2005; 331: 938–39

22. N. M. Hadler, Plaint of the aged worker, *Journal of Occupational and Environmental Medicine* 1997; 39 (12): 1141.

23. A. Kouvonen, M. Kivimäki, A. Väänänen, et al., Job strain and adverse health behaviors: The Finnish Public Sector Study, *Journal of Occupational and Environmental Medicine* 2007; 49: 68–74.

24. W. Poortinga, Do health behaviors mediate the association between social capital and health?, *Preventive Medicine* 2006; 43: 488–93.

25. C. Zwerling, P. S. Whitten, C. S. Davis, and N. L. Sprince, Occupational injuries among older workers with visual, auditory and other impairments, *Journal of Occupational and Environmental Medicine* 1998; 40: 720–23.

26. J. Biddle, L. I. Boden, and R. T. Reville, Older workers face more serious consequences from workplace injuries, *Health and Income Security for an Aging Workplace* 2003; 5: 1–4 (www.nasi.org).

27. M. Karpansalo, P. Manninen, T. A. Lakka, et al., Physical workload and risk of early retirement: Prospective population-based study among middle-aged men, *Journal of Occupational and Environmental Medicine* 2002; 44: 930–39.

28. R.-L. Franche, C. N. Severin, S. Hogg-Johnson, et al., A multivariate analysis of factors associated with early offer and acceptance of a work accommodation following an occupational musculoskeletal injury, *Journal of Occupational and Environmental Medicine* 2009; 51: 969–83; W. IJzelenberg and A. Burdorf, Risk factors for musculoskeletal symptoms and ensuing health care use and sick leave, *Spine* 2005; 30: 1550–56.

29. S. Rietdyk, J. D. McGlothlin, and M. J. Knezovich, Work experience mitigated age-related differences in balance and mobility during surface accommodation, *Clinical Biomechanics* 2005; 20: 1085–93.

30. H. Allen, C. Woock, L. Barrington, and W. Bunn, Age, overtime, and employee

health, safety and productivity outcomes: A case study, *Journal of Occupational and Environmental Medicine* 2008; 50: 873–94.

31. I. Kawachi, Injustice at work and health: Causation or correlation?, *Journal of Occupational and Environmental Medicine* 2006; 63: 578–79.

32. B. R. McAvoy and J. Murtagh, Workplace bullying, *British Medical Journal* 2003; 326: 776–77.

33 P W Stone, Y Du, and R. R. M. Gershon, Organizational climate and occupational health outcomes in hospital nurses, *Journal of Occupational and Environmental Medicine* 2007; 49: 50–58.

34. R. R. M. Gershon, S. Lin, and X. Li, Work stress in aging police officers, *Journal of Occupational and Environmental Medicine* 2002; 44: 160–67.

35. G. M. H. Swaen, U. Bültman, I. Kant, and L. G. P. M. van Amelsvoort, Effects of job insecurity from a workplace closure threat on fatigue and psychological distress, *Journal of Occupational and Environmental Medicine* 2004; 46: 443–49.

36. J. Vahtera, M. Kivimäki, and J. Pentti, Effect of organizational downsizing on health of employees, *Lancet* 1997; 350: 1124–28.

37. Hadler, *Stabbed in the back*.

38. J. Vahtera, M. Kivimäki, P. Forma, et al., Organizational downsizing as a predictor of disability pension: The 10-town prospective cohort study, *Journal of Epidemiology and Community Health* 2005; 59: 238–42.

39. J. Vahtera, M. Kivimäki, J. Pentti, et al., Organisational downsizing, sickness absence and mortality: 10-town prospective cohort study, *British Medical Journal* 2004; doi:10.1136/bmj.37972.496262.0D.

40. M. Bartley, A. Sacker, and P. Clarke, Employment status, employment conditions and limiting illness: Prospective evidence from the British household panel survey, 1991–2001, *Journal of Epidemiology and Community Health* 2004; 58: 501–6; M. Kriegbaum, U. Christensen, R. Lund, and M. Osler, Job losses and accumulated number of broken partnerships increase risk of premature mortality in Danish men born in 1953, *Journal of Occupational and Environmental Medicine* 2009; 51: 708–13; K. Struly, Job loss and health in the U.S. labor market, *Demography* 2009; 46: 221–46; W. T. Gallo, H. M. Teng, T. A. Falba, S. V. Kasl, H. M. Krumholz, and E. H. Bradley, The impact of late career job loss on myocardial infarction and stroke: A 10-year follow-up using the health and retirement survey, *Journal of Occupational and Environmental Medicine* 2006; 63: 683–87; D. Sullivan and T. von Wachter, Job displacement and mortality: An analysis using administrative data, *Quarterly Journal of Economics* 2009; 124: 1265–1306; M. Sinokki, K. Hinkka, K. Ahola, et al., Social support as a predictor of disability pension: The Finnish Health 2000 Study, *Journal of Occupational and Environmental Medicine* 2010; 52: 733–39.

41. David Lloyd George in J. Grigg, *Lloyd George: The people's champion, 1902–1911* (London: Eyre Methuen, 1978), 333.

42. Hadler, *Stabbed in the back*.

43. S. Mattke, A. Balakrishnan, G. Bergamo, and S. J. Newberry, A review of methods to measure health-related productivity loss, *American Journal of Managed Care* 2007; 13: 211–17; J. J. Collins, C. M. Baase, C. E. Sharda, et al., The assessment of chronic health conditions on work performance, absence, and total economic impact for employers, *Journal of Occupational and Environmental Medicine* 2005; 47: 547–57.

44. A. F. Mannion, B. Horisberger, C. Eisenring, et al., The association between beliefs about low back pain and work presenteeism, *Journal of Occupational and Environmental Medicine* 2009; 51: 1256–66.

45. N. Gilbert, *Transformation of the Welfare State* (Oxford: Oxford University Press, 2004), 43.

46. Hadler, *Stabbed in the back*.

47. Studs Terkel, *Working: People talk about what they do all day and how they feel about what they do* (Harmondsworth, UK: Penguin, 1985 [1975]).

48. President Franklin D. Roosevelt, Congressional address, *Congressional Record*, June 8, 1934.

Chapter 5

1. S. R. Cummings and L. F. Melton, Epidemiology and outcomes of osteoporotic fractures, *Lancet* 2002; 359: 1761–67.

2. J. A. Cauley, M. C. Hochberg, L.-Y. Lui, et al., Long-term risk of incident vertebral fractures, *Journal of the American Medical Association* 2007; 298: 2761–67.

3. N. M. Hadler, *The last well person: How to stay well despite the health-care system* (Montreal: McGill-Queens University Press, 2004); N. M. Hadler, *Worried sick: A prescription for health in an overtreated America* (Chapel Hill: University of North Carolina Press, 2008).

4. P. Alonso-Coello, A. L. Garcia Franco, G. Guyatt, and R. Moynihan, Drugs for pre-osteoporosis: Prevention or disease mongering?, *British Medical Journal* 2008; 336: 126–29; G. N. Grob, From aging to pathology: The case of osteoporosis, *Journal of the History of Medicine and Allied Sciences* 2010; doi:10.1093/jhmas/jrq011.

5. P. Conrad, T. Mackie, and A. Mehrotra, Estimating the costs of medicalization, *Social Science and Medicine* 2010; 70: 1943–47.

6. Assessment of fracture risk and its application to screening for postmenopausal osteoporosis: Report of a WHO study group, World Health Organization Technical Report Series 1994; 843: 1–129; J. A. Kanis, Assessment of fracture risk and its application to screening for post-menopausal osteoporosis: Synopsis of a WHO report; WHO Study Group, *Osteoporosis International* 1994; 4: 368–81.

7. J. A. Kanis, O. Johnell, A. Oden, et al., Ten year probabilities of osteoporotic fractures according to BMD and diagnostic thresholds, *Osteoporosis International* 2001; 12: 989–95.

8. J. A. Pasco, E. Seeman, M. J. Henry, et al., The population burden of fractures originates in women with osteopenia, not osteoporosis, *Osteoporosis International* 2006; 17: 1404–9.

9. A. M. Cheung and A. S. Detsky, Osteoporosis and fractures: Missing the bridge?, *Journal of the American Medical Association* 2008; 299: 1468–70.

10. J. A. Kanis, O. Johnell, A. Oden, H. Johansson, and E. McCloskey, FRAX and the assessment of fracture probability in men and women in the UK, *Osteoporosis International* 2008; 19: 385–97.

11. C. S. Colón-Emeric and K. W. Lyles, Should there be a fracas over FRAX and other fracture prediction tools?, *Archives of Internal Medicine* 2009; 169: 2094–95.

12. K. E. Ensrud, L.-Y. Lui, B. C. Taylor, et al., A comparison of prediction models for fractures in older women, *Archives of Internal Medicine* 2009; 169: 2087–94.

13. D. M. Kado, K. Prenovost, and C. Crandall, Narrative review: Hyperkyphosis in older persons, *Annals of Internal Medicine* 2007; 147: 330–38.

14. R. Buchbinder, R. H. Osborne, P. R. Ebeling, et al., A randomized trial of vertebroplasty for painful osteoporotic vertebral fractures, *New England Journal of Medicine* 2009; 361: 557–68; D. F. Kallmes, B. A. Comstock, P. J. Heagerty, et al., A randomized trial of vertebroplasty for osteoporotic spinal fractures, *New England Journal of Medicine* 2009; 361: 569–79.

15. R. Rousing, M. O. Andersen, S. M. Jespersen, K. Thomsen, and J. Lauritsen, Percutaneous vertebroplasty compared to conservative treatment in patients with painful acute or subacute osteoporotic vertebral fractures, *Spine* 2009; 34: 1349–54.

16. P. Noonan, Randomized vertebroplasty trials: Bad news or sham news?, *American Journal of Neuroradiology* 2009; 30: 1808–9; C. M. Bono, M. Heggeness, C. Mick, et al., Newly released vertebroplasty randomized controlled trials: A tale of two trials, *Spine Journal* 2010; 10: 238–40.

17. F. G. Miller and D. F. Kallmes, The case of vertebroplasty trials: Promoting a culture of evidence-based procedural medicine, *Spine* 2010; 35: 2023–26.

18. G. B. J. Andersson, Vertebroplasty: One solution does not fit all, *Nature Reviews Rheumatology* 2009; 5: 662–63.

19. J. N. Weinstein, Balancing science and informed choice in decisions about vertebroplasty, *New England Journal of Medicine* 2009; 361: 619–21.

20. T. S. Carey, Commentary, *ACP Journal Club* 2009; 151: JC6 8–9.

21. A. Qaseem, V. Snow, P. Shekelle, R. Hopkins, M. A. Forciea, and D. K. Owens for the Clinical Efficacy Assessment Subcommittee of the American College of Physicians, Pharmacologic treatment of low bone density or osteoporosis to prevent fractures: A clinical practice guideline from the American College of Physicians, *Annals of Internal Medicine* 2008; 149: 404–15.

22. C. M. Black, P. D. Delmas, R. Eastell, et al., Once-yearly zoledronic acid for treatment of postmenopausal osteoporosis, *New England Journal of Medicine* 2007; 356: 1809–22.

23. S. M. Cadarette, J. N. Katz, A. Brookhart, et al., Relative effectiveness of osteoporosis drugs for preventing non-vertebral fracture, *Annals of Internal Medicine* 2008; 148: 637–46; M. J. Favus, Bisphosphonates for osteoporosis, *New England Journal of Medicine* 2010; 363: 2027–35.

24. E. Shane, Evolving data about subtrochanteric fractures and bisphosphonates, *New England Journal of Medicine* 2010; 362: 1825–27.

25. D. M. Black, M. P. Kelly, H. K. Genant, et al., Bisphosphonates and fractures of the subtrochanteric or diaphyseal femur, *New England Journal of Medicine* 2010; 362: 1761–71; B. M. Kuehn, Studies prove possible link between bisphosphonates and femoral fractures, *Journal of the American Medical Association* 2010; 303: 1795–97.

26. S. Lehrer, A. Montazem, L. Ramanathan, et al., Bisphosphonate-induced osteonecrosis of the jaws, bone markers, and a hypothesized candidate gene, *Journal of Oral and Maxillofacial Surgery* 2009; 67: 159–61.

27. S. R. Heckbert, G. Li, S. R. Cummings, N. L. Smith, and B. M. Psaty, Use of alendronate and risk of incident atrial fibrillation in women, *Archives of Internal Medicine* 2008; 168: 826–31.

28. J. R. Center, D. Bliuc, T. V. Nguyen, and J. A. Eisman, Risk of subsequent fracture after low-trauma fracture in men and women, *Journal of the American Medical Association* 2007; 297: 387–94.

29. A. Qaseem, V. Snow, P. Shekelle, et al., Screening for osteoporosis in men: A clinical practice guideline from the American College of Physicians, *Annals of Internal Medicine* 2008; 148: 680–84; H. Liu, N. M. Paige, C. L. Goldzweig, et al., Screening for osteoporosis in men: A systematic review for an American College of Physicians Guideline, *Annals of Internal Medicine* 2008; 148: 685–701.

30. E. Barrett-Connor, C. M. Nielson, E. Orwoll, D. C. Bauer, and J. A. Cauley, Epidemiology of rib fractures in older men: Osteoporotic fractures in men (MrOS) prospective cohort study, *British Medical Journal* 2010; 340: c1069, doi:10.1136/bmj.c1069.

31. S. R. Salpeter, N. S. Buckley, H. Liu, and E. E. Salpeter, The cost-effectiveness of hormone therapy in younger and older postmenopausal women, *American Journal of Medicine* 2009; 122: 42–52.

32. M. H. Emmelot-Vonk, H. J. Verhaar, H. R. Nakhai Pour, et al., Effect of testosterone supplementation on functional mobility, cognition, and other parameters in older men: A randomized controlled trial, *Journal of the American Medical Association* 2008; 299: 39–52; S. Basaria, A. D. Coviello, T. G. Travison, et al., Adverse events associated with testosterone administration, *New England Journal of Medicine* 2010; 363: 109–22; W. J. Bremner, Testosterone deficiency and replacement in older men, *New England Journal of Medicine* 2010; 363: 189–91.

33. K. Sreekumaran Nair, R. A. Rizza, P. O'Brien, et al., DHEA in elderly women and DHEA or testosterone in elderly men, *New England Journal of Medicine* 2006; 355: 1647–59; P. M. Stewart, Aging and fountain-of-youth hormones, *New England Journal of Medicine* 2006; 355: 1724–25.

34. E. Canalis, A. Giustina, and J. P. Bilezikian, Mechanisms of anabolic therapies for osteoporosis, *New England Journal of Medicine* 2007; 357: 905–16.

35. H. A. Bischoff-Ferrari, W. C. Willett, J. B. Wong, et al., Prevention of nonvertebral fractures with oral vitamin D and dose dependency, *Archives of Internal Medicine* 2009; 169: 551–61; H. A. Bischoff-Ferrari, W. C. Willett, J. B. Wong, et al., Prevention of nonvertebral fractures with oral vitamin D and dose dependency, *Archives of Internal Medicine* 2009; 169: 551–61, with commentary by M. Denman, *ACP Journal Club* 2009; 151: JC2–8.

36. DIPART Group, Patient level pooled analysis of 68,500 patients from seven major vitamin D fracture trials in U.S. and Europe, *British Medical Journal* 2010; 340: b5463, doi:10.1136/bmj.b5463.

37. C. Jackson, S. Gaugris, S. Sen, and D. Hosking, The effect of cholecalciferol (vitamin D3) on the risk of fall and fracture: A meta-analysis, *Quarterly Journal of Medicine* 2007; 100: 185–92; H. A. Bischoff-Ferrari, B. Dawson-Hughes, H. B. Staehelin, et al., Fall prevention with supplemental and active forms of vitamin D: A meta-analysis of randomised controlled trials, *British Medical Journal* 2009; 339: b3692.

38. K. M. Sanders, A. L. Stuart, E. J. Williamson, et al., Annual high-dose oral vitamin D and falls and fractures in older women, *Journal of the American Medical Association* 2010; 303: 1815–22.

39. G. Bjelakovic, D. Nikolova, L. L. Gluud, R. G. Simonetti, and C. Gluud, Mortality in randomized trials of antioxidant supplements for primary and secondary prevention:

Systematic review and meta-analysis, *Journal of the American Medical Association* 2007; 297: 842–57.

40. E. Guallar and E. R. Miller, Vitamin D supplementation in the age of lost innocence, *Annals of Internal Medicine* 2010; 152: 327–29; Committee to Review Dietary Reference Intakes for Vitamin D and Calcium, Dietary reference intakes for calcium and vitamin D, Institute of Medicine of the National Academies, Washington, D.C., 2010.

41. D. Bliuc, N. D. Nguyen, V. E. Milch, et al., Mortality risk associated with low-trauma osteoporotic fracture and subsequent fracture in men and women, *Journal of the American Medical Association* 2009; 301: 513–21.

42. P. Haentjens, J. Magaziner, C. S. Colón-Emeric, et al., Meta-analysis: Excess mortality after hip fracture among older women and men, *Annals of Internal Medicine* 2010; 152: 380–90.

43. C. A. Brauer, M. Coca-Perraillon, D. M. Cutler, and A. B. Rosen, Incidence and mortality of hip fractures in the United States, *Journal of the American Medical Association* 2009; 301: 1573–79; W. D. Leslie, S. O'Donnell, S. Jean, et al., Trends in hip fracture rates in Canada, *Journal of the American Medical Association* 2009; 301: 883–89.

44. T. Järvinen, H. Slevänen, K. M. Khan, A. Heinonen, and P. Kannus, Shifting the focus in fracture prevention from osteoporosis to falls, *British Medical Journal* 2008; 336: 124–26; R. Katz and P. Shah, The patient who falls: Challenges for families, clinicians, and communities, *Journal of the American Medical Association* 2010; 303: 273–74; Y. L. Michael, E. P. Whitlock, J. S. Lin, et al., Primary care–relevant interventions to prevent falling in older adults: A systematic evidence review for the U.S. Preventive Services Task Force, *Annals of Internal Medicine* 2010; 153: 815–25.

45. M. J. Haran, I. D. Cameron, R. Q. Ivers, et al., Effect on falls of providing single lens distance vision glasses to multifocal glasses wearers: VISIBLE randomised controlled trial, *British Medical Journal* 2010; 340: c2265, doi:10.1136/bjm.c2265.

46. J. C. Woolcott, K. J. Richardson, M. O. Wiens, et al., Meta-analysis of the impact of 9 medication classes on falls in elderly persons, *Archives of Internal Medicine* 2009; 169: 1952–60.

47. K. W. Saunders, K. M. Dunn, J. O. Merrill, et al., Relationship of opioid use and dosage levels to fractures in older chronic pain patients, *Journal of General Internal Medicine* 2010; 25: 310–15; M. Papaleontiou, C. R. Henderson Jr., B. J. Turner, et al., Outcomes associated with opioid use in the treatment of chronic noncancer pain in older adults: A systematic review and meta-analysis, *Journal of the American Geriatrics Society* 2010; 58: 1353–69.

48. S. G. Leveille, R. N. Jones, D. K. Kiely, et al., Chronic musculoskeletal pain and the occurrence of falls in an older population, *Journal of the American Medical Association* 2009; 302: 2214–21.

49. American Geriatrics Society Panel on the Pharmacological Management of Persistent Pain in Older Persons, Pharmacological management of persistent pain in older persons, *Journal of the American Geriatrics Society* 2009; 57: 1331–46.

50. W. C. Li, Y. C. Chen, R. S. Yang, and J. Y. Tsauo, Effects of exercise programmes on quality of life in osteoporotic and osteopenic postmenopausal women: A systematic review and meta-analysis. *Clinical Rehabilitation* 2009; 23: 888–96.

51. S. Gates, S. E. Lamb, J. D. Fisher, M. W. Cooke, and Y. H. Carter, Multifactorial as-

sessment and targeted intervention for preventing falls and injuries among older people in community and emergency care settings: Systematic review and meta-analysis, *British Medical Journal* 2008; 336: 130–33; W. J. Gillespie, L. D. Gillespie, and M. J. Parker, Hip protectors for preventing hip fractures in older people, Cochrane Database of Systematic Reviews 2010, issue 10, art. no. CD001255, doi:10.1002/14651858.CD001255.pub4.

52. M. E. Tinetti, D. I. Baker, M. King, et al., Effect of dissemination of evidence in reducing injuries from falls, *New England Journal of Medicine* 2008; 359: 252–61; M. E. Tinetti and C. Kumar, The patient who falls, *Journal of the American Medical Association* 2010; 303: 258–66.

53. H. D. Nelson, E. M. Haney, T. Dana, C. Bougatsos, and R. Chou, Screening for osteoporosis: An update for the U.S. Preventive Services Task Force, *Annals of Internal Medicine* 2010; 153: 99–111.

54. S. L. Edmond and D. T. Felson, Prevalence of back symptoms in elders, *Journal of Rheumatology* 2000; 27: 220–25.

55. H. Verbiest, Fallacies of the present definition, nomenclature, and classification of the stenosis of the lumbar vertebral canal, *Spine* 1976; 1: 217–25.

56. J. N. Katz, G. Stucki, S. J. Lipson, et al., Predictors of surgical outcome in degenerative lumbar spinal stenosis, *Spine* 1999; 24: 2229–33; A. C. Simotas, F. J. Dorey, K. K. Hansraj, and F. Cammisa, Nonoperative treatment for lumbar spinal stenosis, *Spine* 2000; 25: 197–204; T. Amundsen, H. Weber, H. Nordal, B. Magnaes, M. Abdelnoor, and F. Lilleås, Lumbar spinal stenosis: Conservative or surgical management? A prospective 10-year study, *Spine* 2000; 25: 1424–36; S. J. Atlas, R. B. Keller, D. Robson, R. A. Deyo, and D. E. Singer, Surgical and nonsurgical management of lumbar spinal stenosis, *Spine* 2000; 25: 556–62.

57. J. N. Weinstein, T. D. Tosteson, J. D. Lurie, et al., Surgical versus nonoperative treatment for lumbar spinal stenosis four-year results of the Spine Patient Outcomes Research Trial, *Spine* 2010; 35: 1329–38.

58. S. Genevay, S. J. Atlas, and J. N. Katz, Variation in eligibility criteria from studies of radiculopathy due to herniated disc and of neurogenic claudication due to lumbar spinal stenosis, *Spine* 2010; 35: 803–11; P. Suri, J. Rainville, L. Kalichman, and J. N. Katz, Does this older adult with lower extremity pain have the clinical syndrome of lumbar spinal stenosis?, *Journal of the American Medical Association* 2010; 304: 2628–36.

59. R. A. Deyo, S. K. Mirza, B. I. Martin, W. Kreuter, D. C. Goodman, and J. G. Jarvik, Trends, major medical complications, and charges associated with surgery for lumbar spinal stenosis in older adults, *Journal of the American Medical Association* 2010; 303: 1259–65.

60. A. J. Haig and C. C. Tomkins, Diagnosis and management of lumbar spinal stenosis, *Journal of the American Medical Association* 2010; 303: 71–72; E. J. Carragee, The increasing morbidity of elective spinal stenosis surgery, *Journal of the American Medical Association* 2010; 303: 1309–10.

61. R. Chou, J. Baisden, E. J. Carragee, et al., Surgery for low back pain: A review of the evidence for an American Pain Society clinical practice guideline, *Spine* 2009; 34: 1094–109.

62. M. C. Reid, C. S. Williams, J. Concato, M. E. Tinetti, and T. M. Gill, Depressive symptoms as a risk factor for disabling back pain in community-dwelling older persons, *Journal of the American Geriatrics Society* 2003; 51: 1710–17; T. Meyer, J. Cooper, and

H. Raspe, Disabling low back pain and depressive symptoms in the community-dwelling elderly, *Spine* 2007; 32: 2380–86.

63. J. Moncrieff, S. Wessely, and R. Hardy, Active placebos versus antidepressants for depression, Cochrane Database of Systematic Reviews 2004, issue 1, art. no. CD003012, doi:10.1002/14651858.CD003012.pub2; H. E. Pigott, A. M. Leventhal, G. S. Alter, and J. J. Boren, Efficacy and effectiveness of antidepressants: Current status of research, *Psychotherapy and Psychosomatics* 2010; 79: 267–79; M. Haas, C. Groupp, J. Muench, et al., Chronic disease self-management program for low back pain in the elderly, *Journal of Manipulative and Physiological Therapeutics* 2005; 28: 228–37.

64. S. G. Wannamethee, S. Ebrahim, O. Papacost, and A. G. Shaper, From a postal questionnaire of older men, healthy lifestyle factors reduced the onset of and may have increased recovery from mobility limitation, *Journal of Clinical Epidemiology* 2005; 58: 831–40.

65. I. P. Donald and C. Foy, A longitudinal study of joint pain in older people, *Rheumatology* 2004; 43: 1256–60; S. G. Leveille, Y. Zhang, W. McMullen, M. Kelly-Hayes, and D. Felson, Sex differences in musculoskeletal pain in older adults, *Pain* 2005; 116: 332–38.

66. M. C. Wang, W. Kreuter, C. E. Wolfla, D. J. Maiman, and R. A. Deyo, Trends and variations in cervical spine surgery in the United States, *Spine* 2009; 34: 955–61.

67. I. Nikolaidis, I. P. Fouyas, P. A. G. Sandercock, and P. F. Statham, Surgery for cervical radiculopathy or myelopathy, Cochrane Database of Systematic Reviews 2010 issue 1, art. no. CD001466, doi:10.1002/14651858.CD001466.pub3; I. P. Fouyas, P. A. G. Sandercock, P. F Statham, and I. Nikolaidis, How beneficial is surgery for cervical radiculopathy and myelopathy?, *British Medical Journal* 2010; 341: c3108, doi:10.1136/bmj.c3108.

68. C. Lavy, A. James, J. Wilson-MacDonald, and J. Fairbank, Cauda equina syndrome, *British Medical Journal* 2009; 338: b936, doi:10:1136/bmj/b936.

69. Hadler, *The last well person*; Hadler, *Worried sick*; N. M. Hadler, *Stabbed in the back: Confronting back pain in an overtreated society* (Chapel Hill: University of North Carolina Press, 2009); N. M. Hadler, *Occupational musculoskeletal disorders*, 3rd ed. (Philadelphia: Lippincott Williams & Wilkins, 2005).

70. M. D. Chard, R. Hazleman, B. L. Hazleman, R. H. King, and B. B. Reiss, Shoulder disorders in the elderly: A community survey, *Arthritis and Rheumatism* 1991; 34: 766–69.

71. L. J. Badcock, M. Lewis, E. M. Hay, and P. R. Croft, Consultation and the outcome of shoulder-neck pain: A cohort study in the population, *Journal of Rheumatology* 2003; 30: 2694–99; L. Linsell, J. Dawson, K. Zondervan, et al., Prevalence and incidence of adults consulting for shoulder conditions in UK primary care: Patterns of diagnosis and referral, *Rheumatology* 2006; 4: 215–21.

72. L. J. Badcock, M. Lewis, E. M. Hay, R. McCarney, and P. R. Croft, Chronic shoulder pain in the community: A syndrome of disability or distress?, *Annals of the Rheumatic Diseases* 2002; 61: 128–31.

73. C. Lehman, F. Cuomo, F. J. Kummer, and J. D. Zuckerman, The incidence of full thickness rotator cuff tears in a large cadaveric population, *Bulletin of the Hospital for Joint Diseases* 1995; 54: 30–31.

74. A. H. Gomoll, J. N. Katz, J. J. P. Warner, and P. J. Millett, Rotator cuff disorders: Recognition and management among patients with shoulder pain, *Arthritis and Rheumatism* 2004; 50: 3751–61.

75. O. P. Krief and D. Huguet, Shoulder pain and disability: Comparison with MR findings, *American Journal of Radiology* 2006; 186: 1234–39.

76. J. C. Selda, C. LeBlanc, J. R. Schouten, et al., Systematic review: Nonoperative and operative treatments for rotator cuff tears; a comparative effectiveness review, *Annals of Internal Medicine* 2010; 153: 246–55.

77. B. W. Koes, Corticosteroid injection for rotator cuff disease, *British Medical Journal* 2009; 338: a2599, doi:10.1136/bmj.a2599; D. P. Crawshaw, P. S. Helliwell, E. M. A. Hensor, E. M. Hay, S. J. Aldous, and P. G. Conaghan, Exercise therapy after corticosteroid injection for moderate to severe shoulder pain: Large pragmatic randomized trial, *British Medical Journal* 2010; 340: c3037, doi:10.1126/bmj.c3037.

78. E. Thomas, P. R. Croft, S. M. Paterson, K. Dziedzic, and E. M. Hay, What influences participants' treatment preference and can it influence outcome? Results from a primary care–based randomised trial for shoulder pain, *British Journal of General Practice* 2004; 54: 93–96.

79. J. Poole, A. A. Sayer, R. Hardy, et al., Patterns of interphalangeal hand joint involvement of osteoarthritis among men and women: A British cohort study, *Arthritis and Rheumatism* 2003; 48: 3371–76.

80. K. Dziedzic, E. Thomas, S. Hill, et al., The impact of musculoskeletal hand problems in older adults: Findings from the North Staffordshire Osteoarthritis Project (NorSTOP), *Rheumatology* 2007; 46: 963–67; S. Hill, K. Dziedzic, E. Thomas, S. R. Baker, and P. Croft, The illness perceptions associated with health and behavioural outcomes in people with musculoskeletal hand problems: Findings from the North Staffordshire Osteoarthritis Project (NorSTOP), *Rheumatology* 2007; 46: 944–51.

81. R. Joshi, Intra-articular corticosteroid injection for first carpometacarpal osteoarthritis, *Journal of Rheumatology* 2005; 32: 1305–6.

82. J. Chen, A. Devine, I. M. Dick, S. S. Dhaliwal, and R. L. Prince, Prevalence of lower extremity pain and its association with functionality and quality of life in elderly women in Australia, *Journal of Rheumatology* 2003; 30: 2689–93.

83. N. M. Hadler, Knee pain is the malady — Not osteoarthritis, *Annals of Internal Medicine* 1992; 116: 598–99.

84. T. Neogi, D. Felson, J. Niu, et al., Association between radiographic features of knee osteoarthritis and pain: Results from two cohort studies, *British Medical Journal* 2009; 339: b2844, doi:10.1136/bmj.b2844; T. Pincus and J. A. Block, Pain and radiographic damage in osteoarthritis, *British Medical Journal* 2009; 339: b2802, doi:10.1136/bmj.b2802.

85. P. A. Kovar, J. P. Allegrante, C. B. MacKenzie, et al., Supervised fitness walking in patients with osteoarthritis of the knee: A randomized, controlled trial, *Annals of Internal Medicine* 1992; 116: 529–34.

86. J. Niu, Y. Q. Zhang, J. Torner, et al., Is obesity a risk factor for progressive radiographic knee osteoarthritis?, *Arthritis and Rheumatism (Arthritis Care and Research)* 2009; 61: 329–35.

87. M. Fransen and S. McConnell, Land-based exercise for osteoarthritis of the knee: A meta-analysis of randomized controlled trials, *Journal of Rheumatology* 2009; 36: 1109–17.

88. G. H. Gislason, J. N. Rasmussen, S. Z. Abildstrom, et al., Increased mortality and cardiovascular morbidity associated with use of nonsteroidal anti-inflammatory drugs in chronic heart failure, *Archives of Internal Medicine* 2009; 169: 141–49; S. Trelle, S. Reichen-

bach, S. Wandel, et al., Cardiovascular safety of non-steroidal anti-inflammatory drugs: Network meta-analysis, *British Medical Journal* 2011; 342: c7086, doi:10.1136/bmj.c7086.

89. E. Nüesch, A. W. S. Rutjes, E. Husni, V. Welch, and P. Jüni, Oral or transdermal opioids for osteoarthritis of the knee or hip, Cochrane Database of Systematic Reviews 2009, issue 4, art. no. CD003115, doi:10.1002/14651858.CD003115.pub3; B. M. Kuehn, New pain guideline for older patients, *Journal of the American Medical Association* 2009; 302: 19–20.

90. Hadler, *The last well person*; Hadler, *Worried sick*; Hadler, *Stabbed in the back*; Hadler, *Occupational musculoskeletal disorders*.

91. E. Manheimer, K. Cheng, K. Linde, et al., Acupuncture for peripheral joint osteoarthritis, Cochrane Database of Systematic Reviews 2010, issue 1, art. no. CD001977, doi:10.1002/14651858.CD001977.pub2.

92. A. W. Rutjes, E. Nüesch, R. Sterchi, and P. Jüni, Therapeutic ultrasound for osteoarthritis of the knee or hip, Cochrane Database of Systematic Reviews 2010, issue 1, art. no. CD003132, doi:10.1002/14651858.CD003132.pub2.

93. S. Reichenbach, A. W. Rutjes, E. Nüesch, and P. Jüni, Joint lavage for osteoarthritis of the knee, Cochrane Database of Systematic Reviews 2010, issue 5, art. no. CD007320, doi:10.1002/14651858.CD007320.pub2.

94. R. G. Lambert, E. J. Hutchings, M. G. Grace, et al., Steroid injection for osteoarthritis of the hip: A randomized, double-blind, placebo-controlled trial, *Arthritis and Rheumatism* 2007; 56: 2278–87.

95. P. Wilkens, I. G. Scheel, O. Grundnes, C. Hellum, and K. Storheim, Effect of glucosamine on pain-related disability in patients with chronic low back pain and degenerative osteoarthritis, *Journal of the American Medical Association* 2010; 304: 45–52; T. E. Towheed, L. Maxwell, T. P. Anastassiades, et al., Glucosamine therapy for treating osteoarthritis, Cochrane Database of Systematic Reviews 2005, issue 5, art. no. CD002946.

96. N. E. Lane, Osteoarthritis of the hip, *New England Journal of Medicine* 2007; 357: 1413–21.

97. L. Nikolajsen, B. Brandsborg, U. Lucht, T. S. Jensen, and H. Kehlet, Chronic pain following total hip arthroplasty: A nationwide questionnaire study, *Acta Anaesthiologica Scandinavica* 2006; 50: 495–500.

98. A. J. Silman, Forty-six million Americans have arthritis: True or false?, *Arthritis and Rheumatism* 2008; 58: 1220–25.

99. L. Murphy, T. A. Schwartz, C. G. Helmick, et al., Lifetime risk of symptomatic knee osteoarthritis, *Arthritis and Rheumatism (Arthritis Care and Research)* 2008; 58: 1207–13.

100. J. B. Moseley, K. O'Malley, N. J. Petersen, et al., A controlled trial of arthroscopic surgery for osteoarthritis of the knee, *New England Journal of Medicine* 2002; 347: 81–88.

101. A. Kirkley, T. B. Birmingham, R. B. Litchfield, et al., A randomized trial of arthroscopic surgery for osteoarthritis of the knee, *New England Journal of Medicine* 2008; 359: 1097–107.

102. R. G. Marx, Arthroscopic surgery for osteoarthritis of the knee?, *New England Journal of Medicine* 2008; 359: 1169–70.

103. J. E. Dunn, C. L. Link, D. T. Felson, M. G. Crincoli, J. J. Keysor, and J. B. McKinlay, Prevalence of foot and ankle conditions in a multiethnic community sample of older adults, *American Journal of Epidemiology* 2004; 159: 491–98.

104. F. Badlissi, J. E. Dunn, C. L. Link, J. J. Keysor, J. B. McKinlay, and D. T. Felson, Foot

musculoskeletal disorders, pain and foot-related functional limitation in older persons, *Journal of the American Geriatrics Society* 2005; 53: 1029–33.

105. H. B. Menz, A. Tiedemann, M. S. Kwan, K. Plumb, and S. R. Lord, Foot pain in community-dwelling older people: An evaluation of the Manchester Foot Pain and Disability Index, *Rheumatology* 2006; 45: 863–67.

106. S. G. Leveille, J. M. Guralnik, L. Ferrucci, R. Hirsch, E. Simonsick, and M. C. Hochberg, Foot pain and disability in older women, *American Journal of Epidemiology* 1998; 148: 657–65; H. B. Menz, K. P. Jordan, E. Roddy, and P. R. Croft, Musculoskeletal foot problems in primary care: What influences older people to consult?, *Rheumatology* 2010; 49: 2109–16.

107. H. B. Menz and S. R. Lord, Gait instability in older people with hallux valgus, *Foot and Ankle International* 2005; 26: 483–89.

108. F. Hawke, J. Burns, J. A. Radford, and V. du Toit, Custom-made foot orthoses for the treatment of foot pain, Cochrane Database of Systematic Reviews 2008, issue 3, art. no. CD006801, doi:10.1002/14651858.CD006801.pub2.

109. M. Torkki, A. Malmivaara, S. Seitsalo, V. Hoikka, P. Laippala, and P. Paavolainen, Surgery vs. orthoses vs. watchful waiting for hallux valgus, *Journal of the American Medical Association* 2001; 285: 2474–80.

110. J. Kohls-Gatzoulis, J. C. Angel, D. Singh, F. Haddad, J. Livingstone, and G. Berry, Tibialis posterior dysfunction: A common and treatable cause of adult acquired flatfoot, *British Medical Journal* 2004; 329: 1328–33.

Chapter 6

1. D. Hamerman, Toward an understanding of frailty, *Annals of Internal Medicine* 1999; 130: 945–50.

2. C. M. Kilo and E. B. Larson, Exploring the harmful effects of health care, *Journal of the American Medical Association* 2009; 302: 89–91.

3. N. M. Hadler, *The last well person: How to stay well despite the health-care system* (Montreal: McGill-Queens University Press, 2004); N. M. Hadler, *Worried sick: A prescription for health in an overtreated America* (Chapel Hill: University of North Carolina Press, 2008); N. M. Hadler, *Stabbed in the back: Confronting back pain in an overtreated society* (Chapel Hill: University of North Carolina Press, 2009).

4. D. M. Qato, G. C. Alexander, B. M. Conti, M. Johnson, P. Schumm, and S. T. Lindau, Use of prescription and over-the-counter medications and dietary supplements among older adults in the United States, *Journal of the American Medical Association* 2008; 300: 2867–78.

5. T. Higashi, P. G. Shekelle, D. H. Solomon, et al., The quality of pharmacologic care for vulnerable older patients, *Annals of Internal Medicine* 2004; 140: 714–20.

6. R. Voelker, Common drugs can harm elderly patients, *Journal of the American Medical Association* 2009; 302: 614–15.

7. B. J. Edwards, J. Song, D. D. Dunlop, H. A. Fink, and J. A. Cauley, Functional decline after incident wrist fractures — Study of osteoporotic fractures: Prospective cohort study, *British Medical Journal* 2010; 341: c3324, doi:10.1136/bmj.c3324

8. D. B. Reuben, Medical care for the final years of life, *Journal of the American Medical Association* 2009; 302: 2686–94.

9. A. Bowling, Honour your father and mother: Ageism in medicine, *British Journal of General Practice* May 2007: 347–8.

10. See http://www.thehealthcareblog.com/the_health_care_blog/2010/01/comparative-effectiveness-research-and-kindred-delusions.html#more.

11. D. Grady and R. F. Redberg, Less is more. How less health care can result in better health, *Archives of Internal Medicine* 2010; 170: 749–80.

12. J. F. Fries, Reducing disability in older age, *Journal of the American Medical Association* 2002; 288: 3164–65; T. M. Gill and E. A. Gahbauer, Overestimation of chronic disability among elderly persons, *Archives of Internal Medicine* 2005; 165: 2625–30.

13. A. E. Stuck, J. M. Walthert, and T. Nikolaus, et al., Risk factors for functional status decline in community-living elderly people: A systematic literature review, *Social Science and Medicine* 1999; 48: 445–69; D. D. Dunlop, P. Semanik, J. Song, L. M. Manheim, V. Shih, and R. W. Chang, Risk factors for functional decline in older adults with arthritis, *Arthritis and Rheumatism* 2005; 52: 1274–82.

14. M. E. Williams, N. M. Hadler, and J. Earp, Manual ability as a marker of dependency in geriatric women, *Journal of Chronic Diseases* 1982; 35: 115–22.

15. A. B. Newman, E. M. Simonsick, G. L. Naydeck, et al., Association of long-distance corridor walk performance with mortality, cardiovascular disease, mobility limitation, and disability, *Journal of the American Medical Association* 2006; 295: 2018–26; S. Studenski, S. Perera, K. Patel, et al., Gait speed and survival in older adults, *Journal of the American Medical Association* 2011; 305: 50–58; M. Cesari, Role of gait speed in the assessment of older patients, *Journal of the American Medical Association* 2011; 305: 93–94.

16. E. W. Gregg, J. A. Cauley, K. Stone, et al., Relationship of changes in physical activity and mortality among older women, *Journal of the American Medical Association* 2003; 289: 2379–86.

17. T. M. Gill, D. I. Baker, M. Gottschalk, P. N. Peduzzi, H. Allore, and A. Byers, A program to prevent functional decline in physically frail, elderly persons who live at home, *New England Journal of Medicine* 2002; 347: 1068–74; M. Brown, D. R. Sinacore, A. A. Ehsani, E. F. Binder, J. O. Holloszy, and W. M. Kohrt, Low-intensity exercise as a modifier of physical frailty in older adults, *Archives of Physical Medicine and Rehabilitation* 2000; 81: 959–65.

18. B. M. Kuehn, FDA: Antipsychotics risky for elderly, *Journal of the American Medical Association* 2008; 300: 379–80.

19. J. C. Fournier, R. J. DeRubeis, S. D. Hollon, et al., Antidepressant drug effects and depression severity: A patient-level meta-analysis, *Journal of the American Medical Association* 2010; 303: 47–53.

20. E. H. Turner, A. M. Matthews, E. Linardatos, R. A. Tell, and R. Rosenthal, Selective publication of antidepressant trials and its influence on apparent efficacy, *New England Journal of Medicine* 2008; 358: 252–60.

21. M. A. Stanley, N. L. Wilson, D. M. Novy, et al., Cognitive behavior therapy for generalized anxiety disorders among older adults in primary care, *Journal of the American Medical Association* 2009; 301: 1460–67.

22. C. M. Morin, A. Vallières, B. Guay, et al., Cognitive behavioral therapy singly and combined with medication for persistent insomnia, *Journal of the American Medical Association* 2009; 301: 2005–15.

23. I. Nygaard, M. Barber, K. L. Burgio, et al., Prevalence of symptomatic pelvic floor disorders in U.S. women, *Journal of the American Medical Association* 2008; 300: 1311–16.

24. T. H. Wagner and L. L. Subak, Talking about incontinence: The first step toward prevention and treatment, *Journal of the American Medical Association* 2010; 303: 2184–85.

25. P. S. Goode, K. L. Burgio, H. E. Richter, and A. D. Markland, Incontinence in older women, *Journal of the American Medical Association* 2010; 303: 2172–81.

26. P. M. Doraiswamy, L. P. Gwyther, and T. Adler, *The Alzheimer's action plan* (New York: St. Martin's Press, 2008).

27. R. C. Petersen, R. G. Thomas, M. Grundman, et al., Vitamin E and Donepezil for the treatment of mild cognitive impairment, *New England Journal of Medicine* 2005; 352: 2379–88.

28. R. J. Caselli, A. C. Dueck, D. Osborne, et al., Longitudinal modeling of age-related memory decline and the APOE ε4 effect, *New England Journal of Medicine* 2009; 361: 255–63.

29. R. A. Kane and R. L. Kane, Effect of genetic testing for risk of Alzheimer's disease, *New England Journal of Medicine* 2009; 361: 298–99.

30. K. Schultz-Larsen, N. Rahmanfard, S. Kreiner, K. Avlund, and C. Holst, Cognitive impairment as assessed by a short form of MMSE was predictive of mortality, *Journal of Clinical Epidemiology* 2008; 61: 1227–33.

31. N. T. Lautenschlager, K. L. Cox, L. Flicker, et al., Effect of physical activity on cognitive function in older adults at risk for Alzheimer disease, *Journal of the American Medical Association* 2008; 300: 1027–37; E. B. Larson, Physical activity for older adults at risk for Alzheimer disease, *Journal of the American Medical Association* 2008; 300: 1077–79; E. B. Larson, L. Wang, J. D. Bowen, et al., Exercise is associated with reduced risk for incident dementia among persons 65 years of age and older, *Annals of Internal Medicine* 2006; 144: 73–81; J. Verghese, R. B. Lipton, M. J. Katz, et al., Leisure activities and the risk of dementia in the elderly, *New England Journal of Medicine* 2003; 348: 2508–16.

32. M. L. Daviglus, C. C. Bell, W. Berrettini, et al., National Institutes of Health State-of-the-Science Conference statement: Preventing Alzheimer disease and cognitive decline, *Annals of Internal Medicine* 2010; 153: 176–81; B. L. Plassman, J. W. Williams, J. R. Burke, T. Holsinger, and S. Benjamin, Systematic review: Factors associated with risk for and possible prevention of cognitive decline in later life, *Annals of Internal Medicine* 2010; 153: 182–93.

33. C. Féart, C. Samieri, V. Rondeau, et al., Adherence to a Mediterranean diet, cognitive decline, and risk of dementia, *Journal of the American Medical Association* 2009; 302: 638–48; N. Scarmeas, J. A. Luchsinger, N. Schupf, et al., Physical activity, diet, and risk of Alzheimer disease, *Journal of the American Medical Association* 2009; 302: 627–37.

34. See http://consensus.nih.gov/2010/alzstatement.htm.

35. B. E. Snitz, E. S. O'Meara, M. C. Carlson, et al., Ginko biloba for preventing cognitive decline in older adults, *Journal of the American Medical Association* 2009; 302: 2663–70.

36. R. Stevens, *In sickness and in wealth* (New York: Basic Books, 1989).

37. J. Williams, *Congressional Record*, May 14, 1969, S. 5202.

38. R. L. Kane, Finding the right level of posthospital care, *Journal of the American Medical Association* 2011; 305: 284–93.

39. N. G. Castle, Measuring staff turnover in nursing homes, *Gerontologist* 2006; 46 (2): 210–19.

40. R. A. Kane and L. J. Cutler, Comparing nursing home rules yields 10 lessons from 50 states, *Aging Today* 2007; 28: 7–8.

41. M. E. Williams and N. M. Hadler, The illness as the focus of geriatric medicine, *New England Journal of Medicine* 1983; 308: 1357–60.

42. F. Vladeck, R. Segel, M. Oberlink, M. D. Gursen, and D. Rudin, Health indicators: A proactive and systematic approach to healthy aging, *Cityscape: A Journal of Policy Development and Research* 2010; 12: 67–84.

Chapter 7

1. D. B. Reuben, Miracles, choices, and justice, *Journal of the American Medical Association* 2010; 304: 467–68.

2. G. Livingston, G. Leavey, M. Manela, et al., Making decisions for people with dementia who lack capacity: Qualitative study of family careers in UK, *British Medical Journal* 2010; 341: c4184.

3. K. M. Detering, A. D. Hancock, M. C. Reade, and W. Silvester, The impact of advance care planning on end of life care in elderly patients: Randomized controlled trial, *British Medical Journal* 2010; 340: c1345, doi:10.1136/bmj.c1345; M. J. Silveira, S. Y. H. Kim, and K. M. Langa, Advance directives and outcomes of surrogate decision making before death, *New England Journal of Medicine* 2010; 362: 1211–18.

4. N. M. Hadler, Reflections of an American educator at the Japanese bedside, *The Pharos* 1994; 57: 9–13.

5. L. Apatira, E. A. Boyd, G. Malvar, et al., Hope, truth, and preparing for death: Perspectives of surrogate decision makers, *Annals of Internal Medicine* 2008; 149: 861–68.

6. J. P. Parker, Doctor-to-doctor: An essay on end-of-life issues, *North Carolina Medical Society Bulletin* 1996; 47: 8–9; J. P. Parker, Don't just do something, stand there, *Groton School Quarterly* 1994; 61 (3): 29–30.

7. A. I. Neugut and B. Lebwohl, Colonoscopy vs. sigmoidoscopy screening, *Journal of the American Medical Association* 2010; 304: 461–62.

8. S. E. Harrington and T. J. Smith, The role of chemotherapy at the end of life: "When is enough, enough?," *Journal of the American Medical Association* 2008; 299: 2667–78.

9. H. B. Muss, H. A. D'Alessandro, and E. F. Brachtel, Case 15-2010: An 85-year-old woman with mammographically detected early breast cancer, *New England Journal of Medicine* 2010; 362: 1921–28.

10. J. S. Temel, J. A. Greer, A. Muzikansky, et al., Early palliative care for patients with metastatic non-small-cell lung cancer, *New England Journal of Medicine* 2010; 363: 733–42; A. S. Kelley and D. E. Meier, Palliative care—A shifting paradigm, *New England Journal of Medicine* 2010; 363: 781–82.

11. F. T. Bourgeois, S. Murthy, and K. D. Mandl, Outcome reporting among drug trials registered in ClinicalTrials.gov, *Annals of Internal Medicine* 2010; 153: 158–66; J. Lexchin, L. A. Bero, B. Djulbegovic, and O. Clark, Pharmaceutical industry sponsorship and re-

search outcome and quality: Systematic review, *British Medical Journal* 2003; 326: 1167–70; R. Jagsi, N. Sheets, A. Jankovic, A. R. Motomura, S. Amarmath, and P. A. Ubel, Frequency, nature, effects and correlates of conflicts of interest in published clinical cancer research, *Cancer* 2009; 115: 2783–91.

12. A. Yassi, S. Dharamsi, J. Spiegel, et al., The good, the bad, and the ugly of partnered research: Revisiting the sequestration thesis and the role of universities in promoting social justice, *International Journal of Health Services* 2010; 40: 485–505.

13. M. Pfisterer, P. Buser, S. Osswald, et al., Outcome of elderly patients with chronic symptomatic coronary artery disease with an invasive vs. optimized medical treatment strategy: One-year results of the randomized TIME trial, *Journal of the American Medical Association* 2003; 289: 1117–23.

14. E. D. Peterson, Patient-centered cardiac care for the elderly: TIME for reflection, *Journal of the American Medical Association* 2003; 289: 1157–58.

15. S. C. Palmer, S. D. Navaneethan, J. C. Craig, et al., Meta-analysis: Erythropoiesis-stimulating agents in patients with chronic kidney disease, *Annals of Internal Medicine* 2010; 153: 23–33; D. E. Weiner and D. C. Miskulin, Anemia management in chronic kidney disease: Bursting the hemoglobin bubble, *Annals of Internal Medicine* 2010; 153: 53–54.

16. M. K. Tamura, K. E. Covinsky, G. M. Chertow, et al., Functional status of elderly adults before and after initiation of dialysis, *New England Journal of Medicine* 2009; 361: 1539–47; R. M. Arnold and M. L. Zeidel, Dialysis in frail elders —A role for palliative care, *New England Journal of Medicine* 2009; 361: 1597–98.

17. C. K. Cassel, Policy for an aging society, *Journal of the American Medical Association* 2009; 302: 2701–2; C. S. Landefeld, M. A. Winker, and B. Chernof, Clinical care in the aging century —Announcing "Care of the aging patient: From evidence to action," *Journal of the American Medical Association* 2009; 302: 2703–4.

18. W. J. Ehlenbach, C. L. Hough, P. K. Crane, et al., Association between acute care and critical illness hospitalization and cognitive function in older adults, *Journal of the American Medical Association* 2010; 303: 763–70.

19. T. M. Gill, H. G. Allore, T. R. Holford, and Z. Guo, Hospitalization, restricted activity, and the development of disability among older persons, *Journal of the American Medical Association* 2004; 292: 2115–24.

20. J. Witlox, L. S. M. Eurelings, J. F. M. de Jonghe, et al., Delirium in elderly patients and the risk of postdischarge mortality, institutionalization, and dementia, *Journal of the American Medical Association* 2010; 304: 443–51.

21. J. M. Kahn, N. M. Benson, D. Appleby, S. S. Carson, and T. J. Iwashyna, Long-term acute care hospital utilization after critical illness, *Journal of the American Medical Association* 2010; 304: 2253–59.

22. H. Wunsch, C. Guerra, A. E. Barnato, et al., Three-year outcomes for Medicare beneficiaries who survive intensive care, *Journal of the American Medical Association* 2010; 303: 849–56.

23. M. Unroe, J. M. Kahn, J. S. Carson, et al., One-year trajectories of care and resource utilization for recipients of prolonged mechanical ventilation, *Annals of Internal Medicine* 2010; 153: 167–75.

24. W. J. Whlenbach, A. E. Barnato, J. R. Curtis, et al., Epidemiologic study of in-hospital

cardiopulmonary resuscitation in the elderly, *New England Journal of Medicine* 2009; 361: 22–31.

25. T. J. Iwashyna, Survivorship will be the defining challenge of critical care in the 21st century, *Annals of Internal Medicine* 2010; 153: 204–5.

26. J. S. Kutner, An 86-year-old woman with cardiac cachexia contemplating the end of her life, *Journal of the American Medical Association* 2010; 303: 349–56.

27. G. S. Sachs, Dying from dementia, *New England Journal of Medicine* 2009; 361: 1595–96; S. L. Mitchell, J. M. Teno, D. K. Kiely, et al., The clinical course of advanced dementia, *New England Journal of Medicine* 2009; 361: 1529–38.

Chapter 8

1. T. R. Fried, K. Bullock, L. Iannone, and J. R. O'Leary, Understanding advance care planning as a process of health behavior change, *Journal of the American Geriatrics Society* 2009; 57: 1547–55.

2. T. E. Finucane, How gravely ill becomes dying: A key to end-of-life care, *Journal of the American Medical Association* 1999; 282: 1670–72; C. Zimmermann and G. Rodin, The denial of death thesis: Sociological critique and implications for palliative care, *Palliative Medicine* 2004; 18: 121–28.

3. T. R. Fried and M. Drickamer, Garnering support for advance care planning, *Journal of the American Medical Association* 2010; 303: 269–70.

4. S. J. S. Lee, K. Lindquist, M. R. Segal, and K. E. Covinsky, Development and validation of a prognostic index for 4-year mortality in older adults, *Journal of the American Medical Association* 2006; 295: 801–8.

5. T. M. Gill, E. A. Gahbauer, L. Han, and H. G. Allore, Trajectories of disability in the last year of life, *New England Journal of Medicine* 2010; 362: 1173–80.

6. L. Partridge and K. Fowler, Direct and correlated responses to selection on age at reproduction in *Drosophila melanogaster*, *Evolution* 1992; 46: 76–91; M. R. Rose, Laboratory evolution of postponed senescence in *Drosophila melanogaster*, *Evolution* 1984; 38: 1004–10.

7. D. M. Friedman, *The Immortalists: Charles Lindbergh, Dr. Alexis Carrel, and their daring quest to live forever* (New York: HarperCollins, 2008).

8. H.-G. Gadamer, *The enigma of health* (Stanford: Stanford University Press, 1966), 66.

ABOUT THE AUTHOR

Nortin M. Hadler, M.D., M.A.C.P., M.A.C.R., F.A.C.O.E.M. (A.B. Yale University, M.D. Harvard Medical School) trained at the Massachusetts General Hospital, the National Institutes of Health in Bethesda, Maryland, and the Clinical Research Centre in London. He joined the faculty of the University of North Carolina in 1973 and was promoted to professor of medicine and microbiology/immunology in 1985. He serves as attending rheumatologist at the University of North Carolina Hospitals. Medical education has been a focus of his career at UNC and elsewhere. He has lectured widely, garnered multiple awards, and served lengthy visiting professorships in England, France, Israel, and Japan. He was selected as an established investigator of the American Heart Association, elected to membership in the American Society for Clinical Investigation and the National Academy of Social Insurance, and elevated to master by both the American College of Physicians and the American College of Rheumatologists.

The molecular biology of hyaluran and the immunobiology of peptidoglycans were the focus of Dr. Hadler's early investigative career, to be superseded in the 1980s by his fascination with what he initially termed "industrial rheumatology." For thirty years, he has been a student of "the illness of work incapacity"; over 200 papers and eleven books bear witness to this interest. He has detailed the various sociopolitical constraints imposed by many nations to the challenges of applying disability and compensation insurance schemes to such predicaments as back pain and arm pain in the workplace. He has dissected the fashion in which medicine turns disputative, and thereby iatrogenic, in the process of disability determination, whether for back or arm pain or a more global illness narrative such as is labeled "fibromyalgia." He is widely regarded for his critical assessment of the limitations of certainty regarding medical and surgical management of the regional musculoskeletal disorders. The third edition of his monograph *Occupational Musculoskeletal Disorders* was published by Lippincott Williams & Wilkins in 2005 and provides a ready resource as to his thinking on all the regional musculoskeletal disorders.

In the past decade, Dr. Hadler turned his critical razor to much that is considered contemporary medicine at its finest. His assaults on medicalization and overtreatment appear in many editorials and commentaries and three recent monographs: *The Last Well Person: How to Stay Well Despite the Health-Care System* (McGill-Queens University Press, 2004), *Worried Sick: A Prescription for Health in an Overtreated America* (UNC Press, 2008), and *Stabbed in the Back: Confronting Back Pain in an Overtreated Society* (UNC Press, 2009). All have been published in French translation by Les Presses de l'Université Laval / Les Éditions de l'IQRC: *Le Dernier des Bien-Portants, Malades d'inquiétude* and *Poignardé dans le dos.*

Dr. Hadler is a diplomate of the American Board of Internal Medicine, as well as its subspecialty boards, in rheumatology and geriatrics and was awarded the American Board's Certificate for Advanced Achievement in Internal Medicine. He is also a diplomate of the American Board of Allergy and Immunology. He has published scientific papers across this spectrum of disciplines. One of the themes of his work melds the insights of rheumatology with those of geriatrics. His interest in aging and its challenges has led to many important publications over the course of Dr. Hadler's career, papers focusing on many of the topics covered in these chapters. *Rethinking Aging* flows naturally from a career-long interest.

INDEX

Bisphosphonates, 121–24; adverse effects of, 123–24; alternatives to, 124; benefits of, 121–23; introduction of, 112; rise in use of, 112–16

Black Americans, disparities in longevity of, 7, 7

Blood calcium, 125

Blood clotting: associated with cardiovascular surgery, 51; drugs interfering with, 53

Blood pressure (BP), high. *See* Hypertension

Blood sugar: with oral hypoglycemic agents, 34–43; in type 2 diabetes, 34, 35, 38

Blood vessels, effects of aging on, 45. *See also specific types*

Body mass index (BMI): definition of, 14; effect of exercise on, 21–22; and longevity, *14*, 14–18, *17*, 43; "normal," 14

Bone: aging of, 111–12; anatomy of, 111–12, *113*, 123

Bone mineral density (BMD): age-related reduction in, 112; bisphosphonates for, 112–16, 121–24; in medicalization of osteoporosis, 111; as predictor of fragility fractures, 116–18; screening of, 112, 116, 117, 130; techniques for measuring, 112, 115. *See also* Osteopenia; Osteoporosis

Bony spurs, 142, 152

Boomers, as aged workers, 93–95

Bouchard's nodes, 143, *144*

Brawley, Otis, 65–66

BRCA genotypes, 63

Breast cancer: early detection of, 65, 68; metastatic, treatment of, 185, *185*, 188; mortality from, 63–64, 69; overdiagnosis of, 66–67; women at high risk for, 63

Breast cancer screening, 63–69; age at, 63–64; vs. cervical cancer screening, 73–74; vs. diagnostics, 64–65; efficacy of, 63–67; frequency of, 63; language used regarding, 68–69; Medicare coverage of, 10; vs. prostate cancer screening, 76–77; risks vs. benefits of, 63–68, *67*

Breast self-examinations, 64, 68

Brigham and Women's Hospital (Boston), 27, 28

Brinker, Nancy G., 188

Britain: abdominal aortic aneurisms in, 56, 86–87; colorectal cancer screening in, 81; decline in mortality from cardiovascular disease in, 50; life course epidemiology in, 90; prescribed exercise programs in, 24; rationing of care in, 161; socioeconomic status and longevity in, 11; vitamin D in, 125

Brody, Jane, 153

Bunions, 155–57, *156*

Bureau of Labor Act of 1884, 93

Bureau of Labor Statistics (BLS), 93

Bursitis, 141

Butler, Linda, 41

CABG. *See* Coronary Artery Bypass Graft

Cabot Case Record of the Massachusetts General Hospital, 186

Calcium: in blood, 125; in bones, 115; and vitamin D, 125–28

Calcium channel blockers, 47

"CALERIE" trial, 25

Calluses, foot, 155

Caloric expenditure, in exercise, 21

Caloric intake: ways of reducing, 26; and weight loss, 21, 25, 26

Canada: BMI and longevity in, *14*, 14–15; colorectal cancer screening in, 79–80, 83; decline in mortality from cardiovascular disease in, 50; hip-replacement surgery in, 151–52; knee surgery in, 154

Cancer: cures for, 19; discussions about prognosis in, 180–81; early detection of, 68; end-of-life decision making with, 180–89; fear of, 68; making informed choices about, 19; metastatic, 184–88, *185*; prevalence of, by decade, 175. *See also specific types*

Cancer centers, 187, 189

Cardiology, interventional, 50–56, 190

Cardiovascular disease: challenge of profiling risk of, 28, 30; in Crestor trials, 27–32; decline in mortality from, 50, 175; fear of, 68; primary vs. secondary prevention of, 28, 32; problems with

Coronary Artery Bypass Graft (CABG), 51–55, 147

Corticosteroid injections, for shoulder pain, 142

COURAGE trial, 52

Crestor: doubts about efficacy of, 30–33; JUPITER trial of, 27 32; side effects of, 31

Critique of Pure Reason (Kant), 195

CROs. *See* Contract Research Organizations

CT scan, before orthopedic surgery, 139

Cultural beliefs: about end of life, 177; about health, 68

Cultural determinism, 68

Cures, for cancer, 19

Cytopathology, 71–72

Dairy products, vitamin D supplements in, 125–26

Death: biological reasons for, 196–98; dignified, 176; at home, 172–74; inevitability of, 1, 6, 176–78, 198; literature on experience of, 198–200; mystery of, 198; predicting decade of, 175; time between retirement and, 5, 12, 170. *See also* End-of-life decision making

"Death panels," 195–96

Debility, hip fractures as sign of, 128

Débridement, 154

Decision making: about cancer, 19. *See also* End-of-life decision making

Decrepitude, 109–57; of aged workers, 101–2; exercise in delay of, 23–24; fragility fractures in, 110–30; lower-extremity pain in, 144–57; neck pain in, 135–37; pinched nerves in, 137–39; spinal stenosis in, 131–35; upper-extremity pain in, 140–44

Deformity, hand, 143, 144

Delirium, 192

Dementia: causes of, 165; definition of, 165; in frail elderly, 165–69, 192; after hospitalization, 192; treatment of, 165–66

Deming, W. Edwards, 107, 197

Denmark, abdominal aortic aneurisms in, 87

Depression: and back pain, 134, 135; in frail elderly, 164; and social capital, 99–100

Determinism, cultural, 68

Developed world, longevity rates in, 2–3, 3, 49–50

Developing world, longevity rates in, 2

Devices, in orthopedic surgery, 147, 150

DHEA, 124

Diabetes, type 1, definition of, 34

Diabetes, type 2, 33–43; definition of, 34; as epidemic, 35, 36; guidelines for screening for, 33–34, 42; hypertension with, 33–34, 42–43, 49; oral hypoglycemic agents for, 34–43; prevalence of, 35; prevention of diseases associated with, 33–34

Diagnosis of Uterine Cancer by the Vaginal Smear (Papanikolao and Traut), 71

Diagnostics, vs. screening, 59–60

Dialysis, renal, 190–91

Didronel. *See* Etidronate

Diet: and cholesterol, 28; and cognitive impairment, 169; in Golden Years, 25–26; and hypertension, 48, 49; sodium restrictions in, xii–xiii; trials on types of, 25–26; and type 2 diabetes, 34, 35; and weight, 25–26

Digital rectal examinations (DREs), 76, 77

Dignified death, 176

Diphtheria, 89

Disability, in frailty, 162–69

Disability determination, 97, 105

Disability retirement, 102

Disc degeneration, 117–18

Disease: "artificial," 89–90; definition of, 9; frailty as, 159; vs. illness, 9–10; in octogenarians, 175–76; screening as search for, 60; ubiquity of burden of, 9–10

Disease mongering, 111

Distal interphalangeal (DIP) joints, 143, 144

DNA, in biological theories of death, 197

Doctors, origins of term, xv. *See also* Physicians

Doraiswamy, P. Murali, 166

Dowager's hump, 117–18

Downsizing, psychological distress caused by, 102–3

Drucker, Peter, 107

Drugs, in elderly: adverse effects of, 161; falls caused by, 129, 161; number taken, 161; over-the-counter, for joint pain, 149; spending on, 35. *See also specific types*

Drug trials: composite outcomes in, 29–31; conflicts of interest in, 28–29, 32–33, 39–40; for Crestor, 27–32; early stopping of, 31; for hypertension treatments, 47–49; for hypoglycemic agents, 35, 36–42; media coverage of, 32–33; null hypotheses in, 41–42; oversight committees in, 29

Ductal carcinoma in situ (DCIS), 69, 75

Durkheim, David Émile, 97–98

Dying: at home, 172–74; human interactions in process of, 173; literature on experience of, 198–200; physician assistance in, 176; process of, vs. frailty, 160–61

Educational achievement, and longevity, 11

Elderly: growing population of, 1; likelihood of becoming, 2–3, *3*, 59; usefulness of prolonging life of, 3. *See also* Octogenarians

Electronic records, limitations of, 93

Emotion, in breast cancer screening, 64–65

Employment. *See* Retirement; Workers

Enabling state, 104–5

End-of-life decision making, 175–94; acute care in, 191–94; advance care planning in, 178–81, 193–94, 195–96; with cancer, 180–89; with cardiovascular disease, 190; concepts of time in, 195–96; end-of-life care in, 181–83; extending life "as long as possible" in, 176–78; intensive care units in, 176–77; palliative care in, 187; quality of life in, 178; with renal failure, 190–91; resuscitation in, 193–94; role of prognosis in, 180–81, 195–96; with terminal illnesses, 180–83

Endoscopy: in colorectal cancer screening, 80–83; definition of, 80

Epidemiological theories of aging, 1

Epidemiology, social, 90

ERSPC trial, 78–79

Erythropoietin, 190

Essential hypertension, 43–49

Esserman, L., 67

Etidronate, 112, 123

Europe: longevity in, 11; prostate cancer screening in, 78–79; rosiglitazone in, 37, 38. *See also specific countries*

European Heart Journal, 38

European Medicines Agency, 37

Evidence-based Practice Centers (EPCs), 82, 83, 85

Exercise, 20–24; and delay of decrepitude, 23–24; and delay of disability, 163, 168; government guidelines on, 22; health benefits of, 21–23; and longevity, 21–23; vs. physical exertion in workplace, 20; prescriptions for, 24; and prevention of falls, 23, 129–30; U.S. fixation on, 20–21; and weight, 21–24

Exercise industry, 20–21

Exploratory analysis of trial data, 32

Falls: drugs contributing to, 129, 161; prevention of, 23, 129–30; and vitamin D, 127–28

False positives in screening, 60, 66

Fat, in diets, 25, 26

FDA. *See* Food and Drug Administration

Femoral fractures, and bisphosphonates, 123

Finland: bunions in, 156; decline in mortality from cardiovascular disease in, 50; social capital in, 99–100, 102–3; unemployment in, 102–3

Finnish Institute of Occupational Health, 102

Finnish Public Sector Study, 99–100

Fitness, in longevity, 21–23. *See also* Exercise

Flat feet, 157

Flegal, Katherine, 16

Flexible sigmoidoscopy, 80–81

Flow, and social capital, 103–5

Food and Drug Administration (FDA): on antidepressants, 164; on cancer treatments, 187, 188; on cardiovascular surgery, 53, 55; and devices in orthopedic surgery, 147; on hypertension, 46–47; on nonsteroidal anti-inflammatory drugs, 149; on procedures vs. drugs, 53; on rosiglitazone, 37, 38, 42; on supplements, 19; ubiquity of drugs approved by, 10; and vertebroplasty, 118, 121; on vitamin D, 125

Foot pain, 155–57; prevalence of, 146, 155; surgery for, 150

Forgetfulness, 165, 166

Fosamax. *See* Alendronate

Fractures, problems with recovery from, 161

Fragility fractures, 110–30; assessment of risk for, 112, 116–18, 122; bisphosphonates for, 112, 121–24; bone mineral density as predictor of, 116–18; in diagnosis of osteoporosis, 112; as normal aging vs. disease, 117; pain of, 118–20; physiology of, 112, *113*, *114*; prevalence of, 111; and prevention of falls, 129–30; vertebroplasty for, 110, 118–21, *119*; vitamin D for, 125–28, *127*

Frail elderly, 159–74; criteria for proper care of, 191–92; disability in, 162–69; as disease vs. stage of life, 159–60; effects of hospitalization on, 192–94, *193*; institutional care of, 169–74; positive aspects of experience of, 159, 160, 172; unique attributes of, 159–60; vulnerability in, 160–62

FRAX model, 116–17

Frieden, Thomas, 36

Frozen shoulder, 142

Fuster, Valentin, 40–41

Gastroenterologists, 80

Gender disparities, in longevity, 7, *7*

Genentech, 188

Generation X, 94, 95

Generation Y, 94, 95

Genetics: in Alzheimer's disease, 167; in longevity, 6, 197

Gershon, Robyn, 102

Gilbert, Neil, 104

Gillings, Dennis, 41

Ginkgo biloba, 169

Glaucoma screening, 85

GlaxoSmithKline (GSK), 37, 38, 41, 42

Glenohumeral joint, 141

Glucosamine, 150

Glucose. *See* Blood sugar

Glynn, Robert, 30–31

Golden Years, 9–57; abnormal weight in, 14–18; biologic imperatives of, 9–11; cardiovascular disease in, 50–56; cholesterol in, 27–33; and clinical judgment of physicians, 57; diet in, 25–26; exercise in, 20–24; hypertension in, 43–49; importance of community in, 12–13; socioeconomic status in, 11–12; type 2 diabetes in, 33–43

Great Britain. *See* Britain

Great Depression, 105–6

Greece, aged workers in, 97

Gripping motion, 143, *145*

Groton School Quarterly, 182

Hadler, Morris H., xi–xiii

Hallux rigidus, 156

Hallux valgus, 156, *156*

Hand osteoarthritis, 140, 142–44, *144*, *145*, 157

Harm, in lifestyle choices, 19

Harrington, Sarah Elizabeth, 184

Health: of person vs. people, 18; physical, social cohesiveness in, 13; social construction of, 68

Health-adverse behaviors: in disparities in longevity, 7–8, 11–12; and social capital, 101

Health care: clinical judgment in, 57; escalating cost of, 90; origins of profit seeking in, 169–70; rationing of, 66, 161, 188

Health-care reform, 4, 66

Health insurance: common sense in coverage of, 10–11; costs of, 188; financial incentives in industry, 188; national, 73, 161

Health warnings, ubiquity of, 10, 13

Heart attack: challenge of profiling risk of, 28; decline in mortality from, 50,

Invincibility, loss of sense of, 160–62
Iwashyna, Theodore, 194

Japan, end-of-life experience in, 180–81
Jaw, osteonecrosis of, 123
Job insecurity: health effects of, 102–3; in younger workers, 104
Job satisfaction, and longevity, 103–4
Joint lavage, 150
Joint National Committee, 46
Joint pain: assumptions about, 146; in hands, 140, 142–44; in lower extremities, 144–57; in shoulders, 140–42; weight in, 148. *See also specific joints*
Journalism. *See* Media coverage
Journal of the American Medical Association, 18, 65
Judgment: clinical, 57; surgical, 138–39
JUPITER trial, 27–32
Justice, U.S. Department of, 92

Kallmes, David, 120
Karasek, Robert, 99
Keats, John: "La Belle Dame sans Merci," 199; "To Autumn," 198–200
Kerr-Mills Act of 1960, 169, 170
Keynes, John Maynard, 107
Kidney diseases: caused by statins, 31; hypertension associated with, 43–45
Kidneys: age-based diminished capacity of, 44; drug side effects in, 44; failure of, end-of-life decision making with, 190–91; functions of, 44
Knee osteoarthritis, 148, 152–54
Knee pain, 146–54; nonoperative therapy for, 150; prevalence of, 146, 152; surgery for, 148, 150, 152–54
Knee-replacement surgery, 153
Knees: anatomy of, 152–53; resurfacing of, 153
Kolata, Gina, 65
Krauss, Ronald M., 26
Kyphosis, 117–18

Labeling, based on screening results, 60
Labor, U.S. Department of, 93
Lane, Nancy, 151

Language: in breast cancer screening, 68–69; of medicalese, 69; used regarding risk in medical journals, 68–70
Last Well Person, The (Hadler), 4, 27, 36
Lavage, joint, 150
Lawsuits. *See* Malpractice lawsuits
Leg pain, 137–38
Leyland, Alistair, 50
Libby Zion Law of 1989 (New York), 92
Lieberman, David A., 83
Life course epidemiology, 90
Lifestyles, 18–20; exercise in, 20–24; making informed choices about, 19–20; sedentary, 15
Ligaments, hip vs. knee, 152
Lindbergh, Charles, 197
Lindström, Martin, 100–101
Lobbyists, health-insurance, 10
Longevity: in Bible, 6, 8; biological reasons for, 197; BMI and, 14, 14–18, 17, 43; exercise and, 21–22; gender and racial disparities in, 7, 7; genetics and, 6, 197; infant mortality and, 6; job satisfaction and, 103–4; recent advances in, 89–90; social capital and, 98–99; socioeconomic status and, 8, 11–12; U.S. rates of, 2–3, 3, 7, 7, 49–50
Long-term acute-care hospitals, 193
Long term care: continuum of, 170–72; rise of, 170
Lottery mindset, in screening, 60–62
Lower-extremity pain, 144–57; conservative vs. aggressive approach to, 147; coping with, 148–49; nonoperative therapy for, 148–50; prevalence of, 144–46; surgical treatment of, 146–48, 150–57
Low-fat diet, 25, 26

Macrovascular disease: definition of, 34; in type 2 diabetes, 33–34
Magnetic Resonance Imaging (MRI): before orthopedic surgery, 139; for shoulder pain, 141
Malpractice, Medical, Type II, 4, 139, 141, 186
Malpractice lawsuits: over breast cancer screening, 65, 67; over prostate cancer screening, 77

Rosiglitazone, 36–42; cardiovascular complications of, 37, 42; government warnings on, 37, 38; marketing of, 37; mechanism of, 37; trials of, 36–42

Rosiglitazone Evaluated for Cardiac Outcomes and Regulation of Glycaemia in Diabetes (RECORD) trial, 37–38, 42

Rosuvastatin. *See* Crestor

Rotator cuff, 141

RR. *See* Relative risk

Sacks, Frank, 25–26

Salt (sodium): effects of restrictions on, xii–xiii, 48; and hypertension, 48, 49; normal intake of, 48

Sanders, Kerrie, 128

Saturated fats, 26

Saul, Stephanie, 41

Scientific evidence, on benefits of surgical procedures, 138–39

Screening, 59–87; abdominal aortic aneurism, 56, 85–87; bone mineral density, 112, 116, 117, 130; breast cancer, 63–69; cervical cancer, 71–74; colorectal cancer, 76, 79–84; conflicts of interest in guidelines on, 84; criteria for, 60–62, 84–87; vs. diagnostic tests, 59–60; doubts about need for, 60–62; prostate cancer, 74–79; reasons for prevalence of, 60; sensitivity of tests, 60, 85; specificity of tests, 60, 85

Secondary hypertension, 43–44

Secondary prevention, of heart attack, 28

Sedentary lifestyle: mortality risk of, 15; and obesity, 21

Seed trials, 33, 37, 121, 189

Segel, Rebecca, 173

Self-employment, 96

Senate Finance Committee, 38

Sensitivity, of screening tests, 60, 85

Shakespeare, William, xiii–xiv, 198

Sham surgery, 55, 119, 139, 154

Shaw, George Bernard, 84

Shieh, Y., 67

Shoes, 155–56

Shoulder pain, 140–42

Sickness absence, 102, 104

Sigmoidoscopy, flexible, 80–81

Six Sigma, 197

Sixty, population over: biologic imperatives for, 9–11; wellness in, 9, 11. *See also* Golden Years

Skilled nursing facilities, 193

Smith, Bill, 197

Smith, Thomas, 184

Social capital, 98–105; of aged workers, 98–105; definition of, 98; and flow, 103–5; regional distribution of, 98

Social cohesiveness: definition of, 98; importance of, in Golden Years, 12–13

Social construction of health, 68

Social epidemiology, 90

Social medicine, 89

Social Security, 106–7

Social Security Act of 1935, 106

Socioeconomic status: in cardiovascular disease rates, 50; and exercise, 20; and frailty, 168; and hypertension treatments, 47, 48; in longevity, 8, 11–12; and social capital, 98

Sodium, dietary. *See* Salt

Specific Estrogen Receptor Modulators (SERMs), 124

Specificity, of screening tests, 60, 85

Spinal fragility fractures, 110–11; bisphosphonates for, 121; physiology of, 112, *113*, *114*; vertebroplasty for, 110, 118–21, *119*

Spinal stenosis, 131–35

Spine: anatomy of, 112, *113*, *114*; fusion of, 134, 135

Spurs, bony, 142, 152

Stabbed in the Back (Hadler), 4, 97, 105, 132

Stage migration, 185–86

Standard of care, in medicalization, 111

Statins: doubts about benefits of, 27, 28, 53; after heart attack, 28; side effects of, 31. *See also* Crestor

Stead, Eugene, xiii

Stents, in cardiology, 51–56

Steroids: for hand osteoarthritis, 144; for lower-extremity pain, 150; for shoulder pain, 142

Stress tests, 52

Suffering, vs. pain, 119–20